The Internal Family Systems Therapy Exercises

150 Practical IFS Techniques for Healing Trauma, Anxiety, Depression, Relationships, Self-Leadership, and Personal Transformation

Raziya McCarthy and Kerry Luther Harrison

Copyright Policy

The Internal Family Systems Therapy Exercises: 150 Practical IFS Techniques for Healing Trauma, Anxiety, Depression, Relationships, Self-Leadership, and Personal Transformation

Copyright © 2025 by Raziya McCarthy and Kerry Luther Harrison. All rights reserved.

No part of this publication may be reproduced, distributed, or transmitted in any form or by any means, including photocopying, recording, or other electronic or mechanical methods, without the prior written permission of the author, except in the case of brief quotations embodied in critical reviews and certain other non-commercial uses permitted by copyright law.

Educational and Therapeutic Use:

Therapists, counselors, educators, and professionals are granted permission to use the worksheets and exercises with their clients or students in therapeutic, educational, or coaching settings. Worksheets may be photocopied or printed for personal or client use only. The sale, redistribution, or transmission of these materials for commercial purposes without explicit permission from the author is prohibited.

Disclaimer:

The information contained in this book is intended for educational and therapeutic purposes. It is not a substitute for professional mental health advice, diagnosis, or treatment. Always seek the guidance of a qualified mental health professional or physician with any questions regarding your mental health.

ISBN: 978-1-7640190-9-5

TherapyBooks Publishing

2nd Edition

Table of Contents

Preface 1

Introduction 4
    Importance of this Workbook 4
    How to use this Workbook 5
    Examples and Scenarios How Therapists Can Use This Workbook 8

Part 1: Introduction to IFS 15
    Worksheet 1: What Are 'Parts'? 16
    Worksheet 2: Exploring the Self and Its Role 17
    Worksheet 3: Identifying Manager, Exile, and Firefighter Parts 19
    Worksheet 4: Mapping Your Inner System 21
    Worksheet 5: Understanding the Relationships Between Parts 23
    Worksheet 6: Common Internal Conflicts 25

Part 2: Identifying Your Parts 28
    Worksheet 7: Recognizing Dominant Parts in Daily Life 29
    Worksheet 8: Understanding Protective Parts 31
    Worksheet 9: Identifying Vulnerable Exiles 32
    Worksheet 10: Journaling Conversations with Parts 34
    Worksheet 11: Listening to the Needs of Your Parts 36
    Worksheet 12: What Does My Part Fear or Desire? 37

Part 3: Working with Protector Parts 39
    Worksheet 13: Exploring Manager Parts (Organizers, Controllers) 40
    Worksheet 14: Exploring Firefighter Parts (Reactors, Soothers) 41
    Worksheet 15: When Protectors Take Over 43
    Worksheet 16: Offering Compassion to Protectors 45

Worksheet 17: Unburdening Protector Parts 46
Worksheet 18: Creating Safe Spaces for Protectors 47

Part 4: Healing Exiled Parts 49
Worksheet 19: Recognizing Exiled Emotions 50
Worksheet 20: Exploring Childhood Exiles 51
Worksheet 21: Visualizing Exiles Safely 53
Worksheet 22: Unburdening Exiled Parts 54
Worksheet 23: Offering the Self's Compassion to Exiles 55
Worksheet 24: Creating Safe Relationships Between Parts 56

Part 5: Integrating the Self 59
Worksheet 25: Visualizing the Self 60
Worksheet 26: Self-Led Conversations with Parts 61
Worksheet 27: Bringing Calm to Your System 63
Worksheet 28: Leading from the Self in Conflict Situations 64
Worksheet 29: Trusting the Self to Guide Parts 65
Worksheet 30: Rebuilding Internal Relationships 66

Part 6: Advanced IFS Techniques 68
Worksheet 31: Building Cohesion in Your Internal System 69
Worksheet 32: Developing Compassion for All Parts 70
Worksheet 33: Resolving Long-Standing Conflicts Between Parts 72
Worksheet 34: Step-by-Step Guide to Unburdening 73
Worksheet 35: Visualizing Safe Spaces for Exiles 74
Worksheet 36: Techniques for Deep Trauma Work 75

Part 7: Relationship between IFS and Trauma 78
Worksheet 37: Understanding How Trauma Affects Parts 79

Worksheet 38: Identifying Trauma-Related Firefighters 80
Worksheet 39: Exploring Trauma-Related Exiles 81
Worksheet 40: Unburdening Trauma in Firefighter Parts 83
Worksheet 41: Supporting Exiles with Trauma 84
Worksheet 42: Creating Safety Before Healing Trauma 85

Part 8: Practical Applications of IFS 88
Worksheet 43: Applying IFS at Work 89
Worksheet 44: Using IFS in Relationships 90
Worksheet 45: Parts Activation in Conflict Situations 92
Worksheet 46: Recognizing When Parts Take Over 93
Worksheet 47: Returning to the Self in Challenging Situations 94
Worksheet 48: Daily Practices to Maintain Self-Leadership 96

Part 9: Specialized Worksheets for Creative Expression 98
Worksheet 49: Using Art to Express Parts 99
Worksheet 50: Writing Dialogues Between Parts 100
Worksheet 51: Expressing Burdens Through Creativity 101
Worksheet 52: Visualizing the Healing Process 103
Worksheet 53: Creating a Safe Haven for Exiles Through Art 104
Worksheet 54: Journaling as a Form of Healing 105

Part 10: Reflection and Growth 108
Worksheet 55: Reflecting on Progress in Healing Parts 109
Worksheet 56: Journaling Your Growth in Self-Leadership 110
Worksheet 57: Understanding Changes in Your Internal System 112
Worksheet 58: Setting Goals for Continued Healing 113
Worksheet 59: Building a Supportive Internal System 115

Worksheet 60: Creating Daily Self-Led Practices 116

Part 11: Tracking Emotions and Triggers 119

Worksheet 61: Identifying Emotions of the Day 120

Worksheet 62: Trigger Response Worksheet 121

Worksheet 63: Checking in with Parts 123

Worksheet 64: Monthly Review of Healing 124

Worksheet 65: Assessing Shifts in Parts and Self-Leadership 126

Worksheet 66: Healing and Unburdening Journey Tracker 127

Part 12: Addressing Specific Client Issues 130

Worksheet 67: Identifying Parts Triggered by Anxiety 131

Worksheet 68: Soothing Anxious Parts Through Self-Compassion 132

Worksheet 69: Recognizing the Role of Firefighters in Anxiety Management 134

Worksheet 70: Developing Self-Leadership to Manage Anxiety 135

Worksheet 71: Identifying Exiled Parts Connected to Depression 137

Worksheet 72: Exploring the Burden of Hopelessness 138

Worksheet 73: Understanding the Role of Protector Parts in Depression 140

Worksheet 74: Offering Compassion to Exiled Parts with Depression 141

Worksheet 75: Mapping Trauma-Related Parts 143

Worksheet 76: Building Safety Before Addressing Trauma 144

Worksheet 77: Unburdening Trauma-Related Exiles 146

Worksheet 78: Developing a Trauma-Sensitive Self-Leadership Approach 147

Worksheet 79: Identifying Shame-Based Parts 149

Worksheet 80: Understanding the Protective Role of Shame 150

Worksheet 81: Healing Exiled Parts with Shame Burdens 152

Worksheet 82: Replacing Shame with Self-Compassion 153

Worksheet 83: Understanding Firefighter Parts and Addiction 155

Worksheet 84: Mapping the Cycle of Addiction in Your Internal System 157

Worksheet 85: Building Compassion for Parts Engaging in Addictive Behaviors 158

Worksheet 86: Steps for Unburdening Addictive Parts 160

Part 13: Exercises for Self-Compassion 162

Worksheet 87: How to Approach Parts with Compassionate Curiosity 163

Worksheet 88: Journaling Compassionate Conversations with Parts............ 164

Worksheet 89: Using Self-Compassion to Soothe Vulnerable Exiles 166

Worksheet 90: Practicing Self-Compassion in Daily Life 167

Worksheet 91: Balancing Compassion for Self and Parts 169

Worksheet 92: Practicing Compassion for Others Using IFS.......................... 170

Worksheet 93: Reflecting on Past Interactions Through a Compassionate Lens 172

Worksheet 94: How to Bring Self-Compassion into Challenging Situations ... 174

Part 14: Mindfulness and Emotional Regulation 176

Worksheet 95: Using Mindfulness to Recognize Parts' Voices 177

Worksheet 96: Developing a Daily Mindfulness Practice 178

Worksheet 97: Grounding Exercises to Return to the Self 180

Worksheet 98: How to Use Breathwork to Soothe Reactive Parts 181

Worksheet 99: Identifying Triggers in Real Time 183

Worksheet 100: Using Mindfulness to Reduce Emotional Reactivity............. 184

Worksheet 101: Mindful Self-Reflection on Difficult Emotions 186

Worksheet 102: Practicing Emotional Regulation Using Self-Led Techniques 187

Worksheet 103: Recognizing the Role of Parts in Overwhelm 189

Worksheet 104: Self-Soothing Strategies for Overwhelming Situations 190

Worksheet 105: Emotional Regulation for Firefighter Parts 192

Worksheet 106: Journaling Through Overwhelm 194

Part 15: Specialized Worksheets for Therapists 196

Worksheet 107: Helping Clients Identify Their Parts 197

Worksheet 108: Mapping a Client's Internal System 198

Worksheet 109: Introducing Clients to the Concept of Self-Leadership 199

Worksheet 110: Exploring Client's Firefighters and Protectors 201

Worksheet 111: Working with Clients Who Have Anxiety 202

Worksheet 112: Guiding Clients Through Depression Work 204

Worksheet 113: Trauma-Informed Unburdening for Clients 205

Worksheet 114: Building Emotional Safety Before Addressing Trauma 206

Worksheet 115: Step-by-Step Guide to Conducting a Parts Exploration Session 208

Worksheet 116: Helping Clients Offer Compassion to Their Parts 209

Worksheet 117: Creating Safe Visualizations for Exiles 210

Worksheet 118: Techniques for Unburdening During a Session 212

Part 16: Worksheets for Stages of IFS Work 214

Worksheet 119: Identifying Your First Protector Part 215

Worksheet 120: Understanding Firefighters' Roles in Stress Management ... 216

Worksheet 121: Simple Grounding Exercises for Beginners 218

Worksheet 122: Beginner's Guide to Mapping Your Internal System 219

Worksheet 123: Exploring Conflict Between Parts 221

Worksheet 124: Understanding How Exiles Affect Daily Life 222

Worksheet 125: Balancing Multiple Protectors in Your System 223

Worksheet 126: Unburdening Exiles for Intermediate IFS Practitioners 225

Worksheet 127: Advanced Visualization Techniques for Parts Healing 226

Worksheet 128: Complex Trauma Work Using IFS 228

Worksheet 129: Advanced Self-Compassion Techniques for Trauma Survivors 230

Worksheet 130: Integrating Unburdened Parts Into Your System 231

Part 17: Emotional Regulation in Relationships 234

Worksheet 131: Understanding Parts in Relationship Conflicts 235

Worksheet 132: Mapping Parts That Impact Your Relationship 236

Worksheet 133: Helping Each Other Soothe Protector Parts 238

Worksheet 134: How to Lead From the Self in Relationship Conflict 239

Worksheet 135: Identifying Your Parenting Parts 241

Worksheet 136: Recognizing Your Child's Parts 242

Worksheet 137: Using Co-Regulation to Support Children 244

Worksheet 138: Parenting with Compassion and Self-Leadership 246

Part 18: Long-Term Healing and Growth 248

Worksheet 139: Daily Check-In with Parts and Emotions 249

Worksheet 140: Monthly Reflection on Unburdening Progress 250

Worksheet 141: Yearly Review of Growth in Self-Leadership 251

Worksheet 142: Goals for Continued Healing 253

Worksheet 143: Weekly Practices to Stay Connected to the Self 254

Worksheet 144: How to Reconnect with Parts After a Relapse 256

Worksheet 145: Preventing Burnout When Leading from the Self 257

Worksheet 146: Creating a Plan for Continued Self-Growth 259

Worksheet 147: Recognizing Patterns in Your Healing Journey 261

Worksheet 148: Building Emotional Resilience for Future Challenges........... 262

Worksheet 149: Evaluating Your Relationship with Self-Compassion 264

Worksheet 150: Cultivating Gratitude in Your Healing Journey 265

Conclusion.. 268

Reference 272

Preface

Healing is an intricate journey—one that requires patience, self-compassion, and the right tools to navigate the complexities of the human mind. Internal Family Systems (IFS) therapy offers a powerful framework for understanding the different parts within us and how they shape our thoughts, emotions, and behaviors. At its core, IFS teaches us that we are not just a single, unified self but rather a system of different parts, each with its own fears, desires, and protective strategies. Some of these parts work tirelessly to keep us safe, while others carry deep emotional wounds. The goal of IFS therapy is to help us build a **harmonious relationship with these parts**, allowing our true Self to lead with **clarity, compassion, and confidence**.

This workbook was created as a **practical guide** to support individuals and therapists in applying the principles of IFS therapy in a structured, accessible way. Whether you are a mental health professional looking for tools to enhance your therapy sessions or an individual seeking self-discovery and emotional healing, the **150 guided exercises in this book** will help you explore your internal world, recognize and understand your different parts, and work toward lasting transformation.

Why This Workbook?

Many people who begin their IFS journey struggle with **where to start and how to structure their healing process**. This workbook bridges that gap by offering **step-by-step exercises** that take abstract IFS concepts and make them **practical, engaging, and easy to follow**.

For **therapists**, this book provides structured worksheets that can be used in sessions to **help clients engage with their internal system**, process past traumas, and develop emotional resilience. The exercises serve as **guides for self-reflection, emotional regulation, and unburdening**, allowing clients to navigate their inner world more effectively.

For **individuals**, whether working independently or with a therapist, this workbook offers a **self-paced approach to healing**. Each worksheet is designed to be **interactive and thought-provoking**, helping you uncover the hidden dynamics within yourself, connect with your Self, and cultivate inner harmony.

What You'll Find Inside

This workbook is divided into sections that guide you through different stages of the IFS healing process:

- **Understanding Your Internal System** – Learn about the core principles of IFS therapy, including the roles of **protectors (managers and firefighters), exiles, and the Self.**
- **Identifying and Mapping Your Parts** – Use structured exercises to discover which parts are active in your daily life and how they interact with one another.
- **Healing Exiled Parts** – Develop compassionate strategies to **connect with and unburden** parts that carry deep emotional wounds.
- **Working with Protectors** – Learn how to recognize and build a relationship with **manager and firefighter parts**, allowing them to trust the Self and ease their protective roles.
- **Developing Self-Leadership** – Strengthen your ability to lead your internal system with **calm, confidence, and compassion**.
- **Applying IFS in Everyday Life** – Explore practical ways to use IFS techniques in **relationships, work, and personal growth**.
- **Tracking Progress and Reflection** – Use guided exercises to track your healing journey, set goals, and maintain emotional balance over time.

A Journey of Self-Discovery and Healing

This workbook is more than a collection of exercises—it is an **invitation to explore your internal world with curiosity and kindness**. The healing process requires **patience and courage**, but through these guided worksheets, you will learn how to create **a safe and nurturing space for all of your parts**.

Whether you are at the beginning of your IFS journey or have been practicing for some time, these exercises will **deepen your understanding of yourself and support you in finding greater emotional balance**. Through **self-awareness, compassion, and intentional practice**, you can **release old burdens, heal past wounds, and move toward a life of greater clarity and connection**.

As you work through these pages, remember that **every part of you has value, and every step forward is progress**. Trust the process, embrace your Self, and allow your healing journey to unfold with patience and grace.

Welcome to the path of inner transformation.

Introduction

The Internal Family Systems (IFS) therapy model has transformed the way therapists and individuals approach healing, offering a deeply compassionate and effective framework for working with the multiplicity of the mind. IFS views the mind as a system of different parts, each with its own thoughts, feelings, and motivations. These parts are often organized into protectors and exiles, with the Self at the core—a calm, compassionate, and healing presence that can lead the system toward balance and integration.

This workbook, containing 150 comprehensive worksheets, is designed to serve as an essential tool for both therapists and individuals seeking to deepen their work with IFS. Whether you are a professional therapist guiding clients through their healing journeys or an individual on a path of personal growth, these worksheets provide structured, step-by-step processes to explore, understand, and heal the different parts of your internal system. The goal is to support the development of self-awareness, self-compassion, and Self-leadership, key components in transforming emotional pain and fostering long-term growth.

Importance of this Workbook

This workbook was developed to fill a critical need in IFS therapy by providing practical, hands-on exercises that complement the core theoretical framework of the model. While IFS itself is a flexible, adaptive approach to therapy, many clients and therapists benefit from tangible tools that help structure sessions and personal work. The 150 worksheets within this book cover all stages of the IFS process, from identifying parts to unburdening them, healing exiles, and sustaining Self-leadership.

Each worksheet has been thoughtfully created to serve a specific purpose, whether it's helping someone identify their protector parts, guide them through a difficult moment of emotional overwhelm, or reflect on their long-term healing progress. These exercises go beyond simple journaling prompts—they are designed to actively engage users in the process of healing, empowering them to lead from the Self and integrate all parts of their system in a safe and supportive way.

How to use this Workbook

This workbook can be used in a variety of settings, and its versatility makes it a powerful tool for therapists, counselors, coaches, and other professionals working with IFS. It is structured to offer guidance through different stages of the IFS process, providing clear instructions on how to identify and work with parts, how to handle emotional challenges, and how to sustain long-term healing. Here's how different professionals can maximize the value of this workbook:

For Therapists and IFS Practitioners

1. **Enhancing Client Sessions:**
    - Therapists can incorporate these worksheets into individual or group therapy sessions to structure the work they are doing with clients. Whether you are introducing clients to the basics of IFS or guiding them through advanced trauma work, the worksheets provide a clear, accessible way for clients to engage with their parts.
    - For example, when introducing clients to the concept of parts, worksheets such as **"What Are 'Parts'?"** and **"Mapping Your Internal System"** can help clients visualize and better understand their internal dynamics. This brings a tangible element to what might initially feel abstract to new clients.

2. **Supporting Homework Assignments:**
    - Therapists can assign specific worksheets for clients to complete between sessions. This helps clients stay engaged in their healing process even outside the therapy room, reinforcing the work done in-session. For instance, a therapist might suggest clients use the

"Daily Check-In with Parts and Emotions" worksheet to promote regular self-reflection, or the "Unburdening Exiled Parts" worksheet to deepen trauma work between sessions.

3. **Tailoring Therapy to Individual Needs:**
    - The structure of the workbook allows therapists to choose worksheets that align with each client's unique needs and stage in the healing process. A client dealing with anxiety, for example, may benefit from worksheets such as **"Identifying Parts Triggered by Anxiety"** and **"Soothing Anxious Parts Through Self-Compassion"** in the "Addressing Specific Client Issues" section. Meanwhile, clients focused on relationship dynamics can work through the "Emotional Regulation in Relationships" worksheets, such as **"Understanding Parts in Relationship Conflicts"** and **"Helping Each Other Soothe Protector Parts"**.

4. **Facilitating Group Therapy:**
    - This workbook is also highly effective in group therapy settings. Exercises such as **"Exploring Conflict Between Parts"** or **"Balancing Multiple Protectors in Your System"** can be used as group activities where participants reflect on their own parts and share their experiences in a supportive environment. Group members can then benefit from collective insight and shared learning, fostering a sense of connection and community in their healing journeys.

For Coaches and Counselors

1. **Guiding Clients Through Self-Exploration:**
    - Coaches and counselors who may not be certified IFS therapists but still use parts-based approaches can benefit from the structured format of these worksheets. The sections on self-compassion, mindfulness, and emotional regulation provide

clients with concrete steps they can follow to explore their internal world safely.

2. **Helping Clients Build Resilience:**
   - Worksheets such as **"Building Emotional Resilience for Future Challenges"** and **"Preventing Burnout When Leading from the Self"** offer practical tools for helping clients develop emotional resilience. These exercises are designed to foster strength and adaptability, helping clients better manage stress, emotional triggers, and potential relapses.

For Individual Use

1. **Self-Guided Healing:**
   - Individuals who are familiar with IFS or are working alongside a therapist can use this workbook as a self-help tool to deepen their understanding of their parts. The step-by-step nature of the worksheets allows users to safely explore their internal system at their own pace. Worksheets like **"Daily Check-In with Parts and Emotions"** and **"Weekly Practices to Stay Connected to the Self"** offer consistent support and guidance for staying engaged with the healing process.

2. **Tracking Progress Over Time:**
   - Many worksheets are designed to help users track their progress, such as **"Monthly Reflection on Unburdening Progress"** and **"Yearly Review of Growth in Self-Leadership"**. These exercises provide a long-term perspective on healing, allowing individuals to celebrate their growth and set goals for future development.

3. **Maintaining Long-Term Growth:**
   - For individuals who have already undergone significant healing, this workbook offers ways to sustain progress, such as **"Creating a

Plan for Continued Self-Growth" and "Setting Goals for Continued Healing". These worksheets encourage users to remain proactive in their healing journey, ensuring that growth and self-leadership are continuously fostered.

Examples and Scenarios How Therapists Can Use This Workbook

This workbook is designed to provide practical support for therapists as they guide their clients through the IFS healing process. Each worksheet offers a structured exercise that can be integrated into sessions, used as homework, or adapted for group therapy. Below are three detailed examples and scenarios that demonstrate how therapists can use the worksheets effectively to address different client needs.

Example 1: Helping a Client with Anxiety and Overactive Protector Parts

Client Scenario:
A therapist is working with Sarah, a 35-year-old woman who struggles with chronic anxiety, particularly in work and social settings. Sarah's protector parts—specifically, her perfectionist part and anxious manager part—often take over when she feels stressed. These parts push her to overwork, leading to exhaustion, while also making her fear failure or criticism. Sarah has difficulty accessing her Self to provide comfort and calm to these parts, and her anxiety becomes overwhelming.

Therapist's Use of the Workbook:
In this case, the therapist decides to introduce Sarah to the concept of protector parts and how they can be managed more effectively by the Self. The therapist assigns Sarah the following worksheets from **Part 3: Working with Protector Parts**:

- **Worksheet 13: Exploring Manager Parts (Organizers, Controllers)**

- **Worksheet 16: Offering Compassion to Protectors**
- **Worksheet 17: Unburdening Protector Parts**

Session Flow:

1. **In-Session Discussion**:
   The therapist begins by explaining the concept of protector parts, focusing on how Sarah's anxious and perfectionist parts are working to protect her from potential failure and emotional harm. The therapist uses **Worksheet 13** to help Sarah identify her manager parts and reflect on how they attempt to control situations when she feels anxious.
   - **Example**: Sarah is asked to reflect on her perfectionist part's role in her work life. She writes down that this part constantly drives her to meet high standards, even when it leads to burnout. The worksheet guides her to see that the perfectionist part is trying to protect her from the shame of failure.

2. **Offering Compassion to Protector Parts**:
   During the session, the therapist introduces **Worksheet 16**, guiding Sarah through a visualization exercise where she approaches her perfectionist and anxious manager parts with compassion. The worksheet prompts Sarah to listen to her parts' fears and offer reassurance from her Self.
   - **Example**: Sarah writes that her perfectionist part is terrified of being judged, and through the worksheet, she learns how to offer this part compassion by acknowledging its fear and thanking it for its efforts to protect her. This exercise helps her begin to build a relationship with her protectors rather than feeling controlled by them.

3. **Homework Assignment**:
   The therapist assigns **Worksheet 17: Unburdening Protector Parts** as homework. Sarah is asked to use this worksheet to visualize unburdening her perfectionist part, offering it a safe space to release the pressure it

feels. She is also encouraged to practice offering compassion to her protectors throughout the week, checking in with how they respond.

- **Follow-Up**: In the next session, Sarah reports that her perfectionist part felt less intense after completing the unburdening exercise. The therapist continues working with Sarah to maintain this balance, integrating additional worksheets on anxiety management as needed.

Example 2: Supporting Couples in Conflict Using IFS

Couples Therapy Scenario:
John and Rachel, a married couple in their mid-40s, have been experiencing ongoing conflicts about household responsibilities and emotional disconnect. John often becomes withdrawn during arguments, while Rachel becomes critical, feeling that John doesn't care. Both partners have protector parts that dominate during conflicts—John's avoidant part shields him from emotional vulnerability, while Rachel's critical part pushes John to engage, creating a cycle of tension.

Therapist's Use of the Workbook:
The therapist decides to use IFS to help John and Rachel understand their parts and how these parts influence their conflicts. They are given worksheets from **Part 17: Emotional Regulation in Relationships**:

- **Worksheet 131: Understanding Parts in Relationship Conflicts**
- **Worksheet 133: Helping Each Other Soothe Protector Parts**
- **Worksheet 134: How to Lead From the Self in Relationship Conflict**

Session Flow:

1. **In-Session Discussion and Conflict Mapping**:
   The therapist begins by explaining to John and Rachel how parts work in relationship dynamics. They introduce **Worksheet 131: Understanding Parts in Relationship Conflicts**, where both partners identify which parts

are activated during conflicts. Rachel identifies her critical part, and John recognizes his avoidant part.

- **Example**: Rachel writes down that her critical part feels desperate to engage John in conversations because it fears being emotionally abandoned. John, meanwhile, writes that his avoidant part shuts down to protect him from feeling overwhelmed by Rachel's criticism.

2. **Soothe Each Other's Protector Parts**:
The therapist guides them through **Worksheet 133**, where they explore how to help each other soothe their protector parts during conflicts. John realizes that when Rachel's critical part is active, she needs reassurance and connection. Rachel learns that John's avoidant part needs time and space to process emotions without feeling pressured.

- **Example**: During the session, they practice offering soothing responses, with John validating Rachel's need for emotional connection and Rachel giving John space without pushing him. Both write down strategies for soothing each other's parts.

3. **Self-Led Conflict Resolution**:
The therapist introduces **Worksheet 134** to help John and Rachel practice leading from their Self during future conflicts. They learn how to pause and check in with their parts before reacting, using Self-leadership to manage emotional responses.

- **Homework**: The couple is encouraged to use these strategies during their next disagreement and report back. In follow-up sessions, the therapist supports them in refining these techniques, celebrating moments where they successfully led from their Self and soothed each other's parts.

Example 3: Group Therapy for Trauma Survivors Using IFS

Group Therapy Scenario:
The therapist runs a group for trauma survivors, many of whom struggle with unprocessed childhood trauma. The group members often report feeling overwhelmed by emotions and are disconnected from their exiled parts. Many members have developed protector parts that engage in self-sabotaging behaviors, such as avoidance or addiction, to cope with emotional pain.

Therapist's Use of the Workbook:
The therapist uses worksheets from **Part 7: Relationship Between IFS and Trauma** and **Part 4: Healing Exiled Parts** to guide the group through trauma recovery work:

- **Worksheet 39: Exploring Trauma-Related Exiles**
- **Worksheet 42: Creating Safety Before Healing Trauma**
- **Worksheet 23: Offering the Self's Compassion to Exiles**

Session Flow:

1. **In-Session Exploration of Trauma-Related Exiles:**
   The therapist uses **Worksheet 39** to help group members identify their trauma-related exiled parts. Each member reflects on an exiled part connected to a specific traumatic experience. In a group setting, they share their insights, learning from each other's experiences.
   - **Example:** One member shares that their exiled part holds deep feelings of abandonment from childhood, and another discusses how their exile carries the shame of past abuse. Group members find solidarity in their shared experiences of exile.

2. **Creating Emotional Safety for Trauma Work:**
   Next, the therapist introduces **Worksheet 42**, guiding members through a visualization exercise to create emotional safety before engaging with their exiled parts. Group members share how they can create internal safe spaces for their parts, fostering a sense of security within the group environment.

- - **Example**: One member imagines a protective environment where their exiled part can feel secure. Others offer feedback, supporting one another in creating personalized safe spaces.

3. **Offering Compassion to Exiles**:
   The therapist concludes the session by using **Worksheet 23** to help members approach their exiled parts with compassion. Group members practice visualizing their Self offering love and understanding to their exiles, beginning the process of unburdening.
   - **Follow-Up**: In the next group session, members discuss how offering compassion to their exiled parts has impacted their emotional well-being. The therapist continues working with the group on unburdening and reintegration in future sessions.

In these examples, the therapist uses the workbook to structure both individual and group sessions, ensuring that clients engage with their parts in a meaningful, guided way. Whether addressing anxiety, relationship conflicts, or trauma recovery, these worksheets provide a concrete, hands-on approach to IFS therapy that empowers both therapists and clients to achieve deeper healing.

The IFS therapy model is a profoundly transformative approach, and this workbook serves as an indispensable resource for both therapists and individuals. The structured exercises in these worksheets offer a clear, step-by-step process for identifying, exploring, and healing parts, all while promoting the development of self-compassion, emotional regulation, and long-term healing.

Whether you are guiding clients through their IFS journey or using this workbook for personal growth, the exercises are designed to foster deep self-awareness and empower users to lead from their Self. By engaging with these worksheets consistently, therapists and individuals alike will find new ways to navigate emotional challenges, build resilience, and create lasting internal harmony.

Blank

Part 1: Introduction to IFS

These worksheets guide users through the process of understanding their internal systems, exploring the relationships between their parts, and resolving internal conflicts. Each step encourages self-compassion, mindfulness, and emotional regulation while deepening the user's connection to their Self and parts.

Worksheet 1: What Are 'Parts'?

Goal: To introduce the concept of "parts" in Internal Family Systems (IFS) therapy and help the user identify the parts within themselves.

Step 1: Understanding the Concept of Parts

- **Instructions**: Read the following explanation and reflect on how it applies to you.

In IFS, each person is made up of various "parts," or sub-personalities, that take on different roles in our lives. Parts may be thoughts, feelings, behaviors, or aspects of our personality that help us navigate the world. Parts are not the same as the Self—they are often protective in nature and may have developed to shield us from pain, fear, or discomfort.

Step 2: Identifying Your Parts

- **Instructions**: Think about situations in your life where you feel conflicted or pulled in different directions. Write down some of the roles or voices you recognize within yourself.

1. When I feel stressed, I often hear a voice that says:
   - Example: "You have to work harder, or you'll fail."
   - This might be a part that wants to push me to succeed.

2. When I feel anxious, I notice a part of me that:
   - Example: "Tries to distract myself with social media."
   - This might be a part that avoids feelings of discomfort.

3. When I feel sad, I have a part that:
   - Example: "Withdraws from people and isolates."

- - This might be a part that wants to protect me from further pain.

Step 3: Reflecting on Your Parts

- **Instructions**: Answer the following reflection questions.

1. How do these parts show up in your life on a daily basis?
   - Reflection: _____
2. Do any of these parts feel like they are trying to protect or help you?
   - Reflection: _____
3. Are there any parts that feel at odds with each other?
   - Reflection: _____

Step 4: Compassion for Your Parts

- **Instructions**: Take a moment to acknowledge that all of your parts exist for a reason. Reflect on the idea that even parts with behaviors you don't like are trying to protect you in some way.

Write down one thing you can say to show compassion toward a part of yourself:

- Example: "I see that you are trying to keep me safe, even though it's hard for me to understand right now."

Worksheet 2: Exploring the Self and Its Role

Goal: To help the user connect with their Self, the calm, compassionate core that can lead and guide the parts toward healing.

Step 1: Understanding the Self

- **Instructions**: Read the following explanation about the Self in IFS.

The Self is the core of who you are—calm, compassionate, and confident. It is separate from the parts that take on various roles in your life. When you are "in Self," you are able to approach situations with clarity and kindness, without being overwhelmed by fear, anger, or sadness. The goal of IFS is to bring your parts into balance by allowing your Self to lead.

Step 2: Recognizing the Qualities of the Self

- **Instructions**: Reflect on moments in your life when you felt centered, calm, and in control. These are likely times when your Self was present.

1. Think of a time when you felt truly calm and at peace. What was happening in that moment?
    - Reflection: _____

2. How do you feel when you are acting from a place of calm, compassion, and curiosity (the qualities of Self)?
    - Reflection: _____

Step 3: Connecting with Your Self

- **Instructions**: To connect with your Self, try a simple breathing exercise. Sit in a quiet space, close your eyes, and take a few deep breaths. Imagine that with each breath, you are inviting your calm and compassionate Self to step forward.

Write down how you feel after doing this exercise:

- Reflection: _____

Step 4: Leading from the Self

- **Instructions**: Think of a situation where you normally feel stressed or overwhelmed by your parts. Write down how you can approach the situation from your Self instead.

1. The situation: _____

2. How can you approach this situation with more calm, curiosity, or compassion?

    o Reflection: _____

Worksheet 3: Identifying Manager, Exile, and Firefighter Parts

Goal: To help the user identify the different types of parts within the IFS model—managers, exiles, and firefighters—and understand their roles.

Step 1: Understanding Manager, Exile, and Firefighter Parts

- **Instructions**: Read the following descriptions of the three types of parts in IFS.

1. **Manager Parts**: These are proactive parts that try to control your life to keep you safe. They may be critical, perfectionistic, or controlling. Their goal is to prevent pain by keeping things under control.

2. **Exile Parts**: These parts hold painful emotions or memories that you have tried to push away. They often carry feelings of shame, fear, or sadness. Exiles are hidden away because the pain they hold is overwhelming.

3. **Firefighter Parts**: Firefighters react when an exile's pain is triggered. They try to put out emotional "fires" by using distraction, avoidance, or numbing behaviors (e.g., overeating, addiction, or shutting down).

Step 2: Identifying Your Manager Parts

- **Instructions**: Think about areas in your life where you feel the need for control or where you hear critical voices. Write down a few manager parts you've identified.

1. What does my manager part say when I feel the need to control something?
    - Example: "I have to stay on top of everything, or something bad will happen."
    - This part may want to prevent chaos.

Step 3: Identifying Your Exile Parts

- **Instructions**: Reflect on moments when you feel sadness, shame, or fear. These feelings might be connected to your exiles.

1. When do I feel emotions that I try to avoid or hide?
    - Example: "I feel a deep sense of shame when I think about past failures."

Step 4: Identifying Your Firefighter Parts

- **Instructions**: Think about ways you cope when strong emotions arise. These coping strategies might be your firefighter parts.

1. How do I react when I feel overwhelmed by emotions?
    - Example: "I distract myself with television when I feel anxious."

Step 5: Mapping Your Parts

- **Instructions**: Now that you've identified a few parts, create a map of your internal system. Draw circles to represent each part (manager, exile, firefighter) and write down their roles.
- Example: My manager part tries to prevent failure by overworking.
- Example: My firefighter part distracts me with food when I feel ashamed.
- Example: My exile holds the sadness of feeling rejected as a child.

Worksheet 4: Mapping Your Inner System

Goal: To help the user visualize and map out their internal system of parts, gaining clarity on how their parts interact and influence their emotions and behaviors.

Step 1: Understanding Your Internal System

- **Instructions**: Read the explanation below to understand the concept of your inner system.

In IFS, your internal system consists of different parts that have their own roles, feelings, and perspectives. These parts interact with one another, sometimes in harmony and sometimes in conflict. Mapping your inner system helps you see how these parts influence your behaviors and emotions in various situations.

Step 2: Identifying Key Parts in Your System

- **Instructions**: Start by identifying a few key parts that seem most active in your life right now. These could be manager, exile, or firefighter parts.

1. **Manager Parts**:
    - Example: A part that controls your schedule or makes you stay organized.
    - My manager part is: _____

2. **Exile Parts**:
    - Example: A part that feels shame or sadness and is often hidden.
    - My exile part is: _____

3. **Firefighter Parts**:
    - Example: A part that distracts you or uses avoidance when you feel emotional pain.

- My firefighter part is: _____

Step 3: Mapping the Relationships Between Parts

- **Instructions**: Draw a visual map of your inner system. Write the names or characteristics of your identified parts inside circles, and use lines or arrows to show how they interact. Think about how each part influences the other.

Example:

- My manager part tries to prevent the exile from feeling pain by being over-controlling.
- My firefighter part steps in to distract me when my exile part's pain starts to surface.

Visual Map:

- [Draw a simple map showing the parts and their interactions.]

Step 4: Reflection

- **Instructions**: Reflect on your map. Answer the following questions:

1. Which part seems to be the most dominant in your daily life?
   - Reflection: _____
2. How do these parts affect one another?
   - Reflection: _____
3. How does mapping your internal system help you understand yourself better?
   - Reflection: _____

Step 5: Building Compassion for Your System

- **Instructions**: As you reflect on your inner system, try to approach each part with compassion. Acknowledge that each part is playing an important role, even if it sometimes causes distress.

Write down one thing you can say to show compassion toward one of your parts:

- Example: "Thank you for trying to keep me safe, even when your methods feel overwhelming."

Worksheet 5: Understanding the Relationships Between Parts
Goal: To explore how different parts within your internal system interact, create harmony or conflict, and impact your overall well-being.

Step 1: Recognizing Interactions Between Parts

- **Instructions**: Read the following explanation to understand the dynamics between your parts.

In IFS, parts are not isolated; they have relationships with one another. Some parts work together, while others may be in conflict. For example, a manager part may try to keep an exile's pain hidden, while a firefighter part steps in to distract you when the pain becomes too overwhelming. Understanding how your parts interact is key to fostering balance and harmony within your system.

Step 2: Exploring the Relationships

- **Instructions**: Think about a situation where you experienced internal conflict. Identify the parts that were involved and how they interacted with each other.

1. What was the situation?
    - Example: "I had to make a difficult decision at work."

2. Which parts were involved?

- Example: "My manager part wanted me to be perfect, but my exile part felt scared of failure."

3. How did the parts interact in this situation?
    - Example: "My manager part took over and pushed me to overwork, while my exile part felt ignored."

Step 3: Identifying Supportive Relationships

- **Instructions**: While parts can conflict, they can also support each other. Reflect on a time when your parts worked together in harmony.

1. What was the situation where your parts worked together?
    - Example: "I had a peaceful day where I felt calm and productive."

2. Which parts were involved, and how did they support each other?
    - Example: "My manager part helped me stay focused, and my Self was able to lead with calmness."

Step 4: Understanding Conflicting Relationships

- **Instructions**: Conflicts between parts are common. Reflect on a recent conflict between your parts and try to understand the underlying motivations.

1. Describe the conflict between your parts:
    - Example: "My manager part wants me to push harder, but my firefighter part wants to distract me with TV when I feel tired."

2. What are the motivations behind each part's behavior?
    - Example: "My manager part is afraid of failure, and my firefighter part is trying to protect me from burnout."

3. What can your Self do to mediate between these parts?

- Reflection: _____

Step 5: Creating Harmony

- **Instructions**: Based on your reflections, write down one action you can take to help create more harmony between your parts.

- **Example**: "I will remind my manager part to take breaks and reassure my firefighter part that it doesn't need to take over."

Worksheet 6: Common Internal Conflicts

Goal: To help the user identify common internal conflicts, understand their root causes, and explore ways to resolve these conflicts using Self-leadership.

Step 1: Recognizing Common Conflicts

- **Instructions**: Many people experience internal conflicts when different parts have competing goals or needs. These conflicts often create tension or stress. Below are a few common examples of internal conflicts in IFS.

1. **Conflict Between Manager and Exile Parts**:
    - Example: "My manager part is constantly pushing me to achieve, but my exile part feels scared and wants to hide."

2. **Conflict Between Manager and Firefighter Parts**:
    - Example: "My manager part wants me to stay in control, but my firefighter part tries to numb my emotions when they get too strong."

Step 2: Identifying Your Own Internal Conflicts

- **Instructions**: Reflect on an internal conflict you've experienced recently. Write down the details of the conflict and the parts involved.

1. What was the conflict?
   - Example: "I felt torn between working hard and taking a break."
2. Which parts were involved, and what were their roles?
   - Example: "My manager part wanted to keep working, but my firefighter part was exhausted and wanted to rest."
3. What emotions did you experience during this conflict?
   - Reflection: _____

Step 3: Understanding the Root of the Conflict

- **Instructions**: Internal conflicts usually have deeper roots. Each part has a reason for acting the way it does. Try to understand the deeper motivations of the parts involved in your conflict.

1. What is your manager part trying to achieve or protect?
   - Example: "My manager part is afraid of failure."
2. What is your firefighter part trying to protect you from?
   - Example: "My firefighter part is afraid of burnout."

Step 4: Using Self-Leadership to Resolve Conflict

- **Instructions**: Self-leadership involves approaching your parts with compassion and curiosity. Think about how your Self can step in to mediate the conflict between your parts.

1. What can your Self say to the manager part to soothe its concerns?
   - Example: "I understand that you want to prevent failure, but it's okay to rest."
2. What can your Self say to the firefighter part to reassure it?

- Example: "I know you're tired, and I will help you find healthy ways to rest."

Step 5: Finding a Balanced Solution

- **Instructions**: Write down a balanced solution that honors the needs of both parts. This should be a compromise that supports both the manager and firefighter.

- Example: "I will take a short break to rest, and then I will return to work with renewed energy."

Part 2: Identifying Your Parts

These worksheets are designed to help users identify their primary parts, understand their roles, and build compassionate relationships with them. By exploring the fears, desires, and needs of each part, users can foster healing and emotional regulation while strengthening their connection to their internal system.

Worksheet 7: Recognizing Dominant Parts in Daily Life

Goal: To help the user identify the most dominant parts that show up in their daily life, bringing awareness to how these parts influence their thoughts, emotions, and behaviors.

Step 1: Understanding Dominant Parts

- **Instructions**: Read the explanation below to understand dominant parts.

Dominant parts are the most active parts in your daily life. These parts often take control in specific situations, guiding your reactions, decisions, and emotional responses. Some dominant parts may help you stay organized or push you to achieve, while others may act to protect you from difficult emotions.

Step 2: Identifying Your Dominant Parts

- **Instructions**: Think about different areas of your life (work, relationships, personal time) and write down the parts that are most active in each of these areas.

1. **Work:**
    - Which part is most active at work?
    - Example: "My perfectionist part shows up and pushes me to work long hours."
    - My dominant part at work is: _____

2. **Relationships:**
    - Which part is most active in your relationships?

- o Example: "My caretaker part takes over and makes sure everyone else is okay."
- o My dominant part in relationships is: _____

3. **Personal Time**:
   - o Which part is most active when you're alone?
   - o Example: "My critical part shows up and makes me feel guilty for not being productive."
   - o My dominant part in personal time is: _____

Step 3: Reflecting on Dominant Parts

- **Instructions**: Reflect on how these parts affect your daily life.

1. What are the benefits of these dominant parts?
   - o Reflection: _____
2. How might these parts cause challenges or stress?
   - o Reflection: _____

Step 4: Offering Compassion to Dominant Parts

- **Instructions**: Take a moment to show compassion to these parts, acknowledging that they are trying to help you in some way.

Write down one thing you can say to offer kindness to a dominant part:

- Example: "I see that you are working hard to protect me, and I appreciate your efforts."

Worksheet 8: Understanding Protective Parts

Goal: To help the user explore and understand their protective parts, which play key roles in shielding them from emotional pain or discomfort.

Step 1: Understanding Protective Parts

- **Instructions**: Read the following explanation.

Protective parts, also known as manager or firefighter parts, work to prevent pain or emotional discomfort. They may show up as critical voices, perfectionism, avoidance, or behaviors like numbing and distraction. While their actions might feel overwhelming or controlling, protective parts are ultimately trying to help you feel safe.

Step 2: Identifying Your Protective Parts

- **Instructions**: Reflect on situations where you felt the need to protect yourself emotionally. Write down the protective parts you notice in these situations.

1. **Criticizing Yourself**:
    - When do you notice a critical voice?
    - Example: "My critical part shows up when I make a mistake."
    - My protective part here is: _____

2. **Avoiding Painful Emotions**:
    - What behaviors do you use to avoid emotional pain?
    - Example: "I often distract myself with TV when I feel sad."
    - My protective part here is: _____

3. **Perfectionism or Control**:
   - When do you feel the need to be perfect or in control?
   - Example: "I push myself to be perfect at work to avoid criticism."
   - My protective part here is: _____

Step 3: Exploring the Motivation of Protective Parts

- **Instructions**: Protective parts often have strong motivations to keep you safe. Reflect on the reasons your protective parts act the way they do.

1. What is your critical part trying to protect you from?
   - Reflection: _____
2. What is your part that seeks distractions trying to avoid?
   - Reflection: _____

Step 4: Offering Compassion to Protective Parts

- **Instructions**: Take a moment to acknowledge the protective role these parts play and offer them kindness.

Write down something you can say to a protective part:

- Example: "I see that you are trying to protect me from pain, and I appreciate that."

Worksheet 9: Identifying Vulnerable Exiles

Goal: To help the user identify their vulnerable exiles, the parts of them that carry painful emotions or experiences, and explore the needs of these parts.

Step 1: Understanding Exiles

- **Instructions**: Read the explanation below.

Exiles are parts of you that carry deep emotional pain, often from past experiences. These parts are usually hidden or "exiled" because their feelings of shame, fear, sadness, or vulnerability are too overwhelming. However, these parts need attention and healing to release their burdens.

Step 2: Identifying Your Exiles

- **Instructions**: Think about moments when you felt intense sadness, fear, or shame. These feelings may be connected to your exiles. Write down the emotions or experiences that these parts hold.

1. **Sadness**:
    - When do you feel deep sadness or grief?
    - Example: "I feel sad when I think about losing a loved one."
    - My exile part holds the emotion of:
    _____

2. **Fear**:
    - When do you feel a strong sense of fear or anxiety?
    - Example: "I feel scared when I think about failing."
    - My exile part holds the emotion of:
    _____

3. **Shame**:
    - When do you feel ashamed or unworthy?
    - Example: "I feel shame when I remember being criticized as a child."

- My exile part holds the emotion of:
  _____

Step 3: Exploring the Needs of Your Exiles

- **Instructions**: Your exiles need compassion, safety, and healing. Reflect on what these vulnerable parts might need from you.

1. What does your sad exile need to feel safe or supported?
   - Reflection: _____
2. What does your fearful exile need to feel reassured?
   - Reflection: _____
3. What does your exiled part that holds shame need to feel worthy?
   - Reflection: _____

Step 4: Offering Compassion to Your Exiles

- **Instructions**: Take a moment to acknowledge the pain that your exiles hold and offer them kindness and care.

Write down one thing you can say to comfort a vulnerable exile:

- Example: "I see your sadness, and I will stay with you as you heal."

Building a Relationship with Parts

Worksheet 10: Journaling Conversations with Parts

Goal: To guide the user in building a relationship with their parts by journaling dialogues, allowing them to understand the perspectives and needs of each part.

Step 1: Creating a Safe Space for Dialogue

- **Instructions**: Find a quiet place where you can reflect. Imagine that you are inviting one of your parts to speak with you. Choose a part that feels prominent or one you would like to understand better.

1. Which part would you like to talk to?
   - Example: "My perfectionist part that pushes me to work hard."
2. What does this part need to feel safe in this conversation?
   - Reflection: _____

Step 2: Journaling the Conversation

- **Instructions**: Begin a dialogue with your part. Write down what your part is saying, and respond from a place of curiosity and compassion.

1. **Part**: "I need you to keep working harder. There's too much at stake."
   Self: "I hear that you're worried about something. What are you afraid might happen?"
2. **Part**: "I'm afraid that if you don't keep pushing, everything will fall apart."

- Continue the conversation, allowing your part to express its feelings and concerns.

Step 3: Reflecting on the Conversation

- **Instructions**: Reflect on the conversation. What did you learn from your part? How can you show understanding or support?

1. What insights did you gain from this dialogue?
   - Reflection: _____
2. How can you support or reassure this part moving forward?

- o   Reflection: _____

Worksheet 11: Listening to the Needs of Your Parts

Goal: To help the user understand the deeper needs of their parts and respond with compassion.

Step 1: Identifying the Needs of a Part

- **Instructions**: Choose one part that you want to explore. Reflect on its behaviors and emotions. What might this part need from you?

1. Which part are you exploring?
   - o   Example: "My anxious part that worries about everything."
2. What does this part do or say when it shows up?
   - o   Reflection: _____

Step 2: Listening to Its Needs

- **Instructions**: Sit quietly and ask your part, "What do you need from me?" Listen closely for the answer.

1. What does this part need to feel safe or supported?
   - o   Reflection: _____
2. How can you meet this part's needs in a healthy way?
   - o   Reflection: _____

Step 3: Offering Compassion and Reassurance

- **Instructions**: Take a moment to offer compassion to your part and reassure it that you are there to help.

Write down something you can say to your part to offer support:

- Example: "I hear that you need reassurance, and I will remind you that you are safe."

Worksheet 12: What Does My Part Fear or Desire?

Goal: To help the user explore the underlying fears and desires of their parts, creating a deeper understanding of their motivations.

Step 1: Identifying the Fears of Your Part

- **Instructions**: Choose a part that often feels strong emotions or drives your behaviors. Reflect on what this part might be afraid of.

1. Which part are you exploring?
    - Example: "My fearful part that avoids taking risks."
2. What is this part afraid might happen?
    - Reflection: _____

Step 2: Exploring the Desires of Your Part

- **Instructions**: Beyond fear, parts often have deep desires or longings. Ask your part what it truly desires or hopes for.

1. What does this part desire or long for?
    - Reflection: _____

Step 3: Balancing Fears and Desires

- **Instructions**: Reflect on how your part's fears and desires are connected. How can you help this part feel safe while also moving toward what it desires?

1. How can you support this part in balancing its fears and desires?
    - Reflection: _____

Part 3: Working with Protector Parts

These worksheets are designed to help users understand, soothe, and unburden their protector parts. By offering compassion, inviting protectors to rest, and creating safe spaces, users can foster balance in their internal system while allowing their protectors to feel supported and cared for.

Worksheet 13: Exploring Manager Parts (Organizers, Controllers)

Goal: To help the user explore their manager parts, which work to keep things under control and prevent emotional distress.

Step 1: Understanding Manager Parts

- **Instructions**: Read the following description.

Manager parts are often highly organized, controlling, or perfectionistic. They are proactive protectors, trying to prevent painful emotions or memories from surfacing by keeping everything in order. While their intentions are protective, they may create stress or pressure by demanding perfection or control.

Step 2: Identifying Your Manager Parts

- **Instructions**: Think about situations where you feel the need to control or organize everything. These might be moments when your manager parts are active.

1. **Control**:
    - When do you feel a strong need to control things around you?
    - Example: "I feel the need to control my schedule completely to avoid mistakes."
    - My manager part here is: _____

2. **Perfectionism**:
    - When do you push yourself to be perfect?
    - Example: "I work hard to perfect every detail at work."
    - My manager part here is: _____

3. **Organizing and Planning**:
    - When do you feel compelled to plan everything?
    - Example: "I make detailed plans to avoid uncertainty or failure."
    - My manager part here is: _____

Step 3: Reflecting on the Role of Manager Parts

- **Instructions**: Reflect on how these manager parts affect your daily life.

1. How do these parts help you feel safe or in control?
    - Reflection: _____
2. How might these parts cause stress or pressure?
    - Reflection: _____

Step 4: Building a Relationship with Your Manager Parts

- **Instructions**: Write down one compassionate statement that you can say to your manager parts to acknowledge their efforts and reassure them.
- Example: "I see how hard you work to keep things under control, and I appreciate your efforts."

Worksheet 14: Exploring Firefighter Parts (Reactors, Soothers)

Goal: To help the user understand their firefighter parts, which react when emotional pain is triggered, often using distraction or numbing behaviors to soothe distress.

Step 1: Understanding Firefighter Parts

- **Instructions**: Read the explanation below.

Firefighter parts are reactive protectors. When emotions become overwhelming or an exile's pain is triggered, firefighter parts step in to "put out the fire." They often do this by using distraction, avoidance, or numbing behaviors, such as overeating, substance use, or zoning out. Firefighters are trying to soothe or calm you, but their methods might lead to unhealthy coping strategies.

Step 2: Identifying Your Firefighter Parts

- **Instructions**: Reflect on moments when you react to stress or emotional pain. These are times when your firefighter parts may be active.

1. **Distraction**:
    - How do you distract yourself when you feel emotional pain?
    - Example: "I distract myself by scrolling through social media when I feel stressed."
    - My firefighter part here is: _____

2. **Numbing or Avoidance**:
    - When do you use numbing or avoidance to cope?
    - Example: "I eat junk food to avoid feeling anxious."
    - My firefighter part here is: _____

3. **Quick Fixes or Reactivity**:
    - How do you try to quickly soothe intense emotions?
    - Example: "I often binge-watch TV to stop thinking about painful experiences."
    - My firefighter part here is: _____

Step 3: Reflecting on the Role of Firefighter Parts

- **Instructions**: Reflect on the impact these firefighter parts have on your well-being.

1. How do these parts help you manage overwhelming emotions?
    - Reflection: _____
2. How might these parts create new challenges or unhealthy coping behaviors?
    - Reflection: _____

Step 4: Showing Compassion to Firefighter Parts

- **Instructions**: Write down something you can say to offer compassion and understanding to your firefighter parts.
- Example: "I see that you're trying to protect me from pain, and I understand why you use distractions to help me cope."

Worksheet 15: When Protectors Take Over

Goal: To help the user recognize when protector parts take over, preventing the Self from leading, and to explore ways to regain balance in their system.

Step 1: Recognizing When Protectors Take Over

- **Instructions**: Reflect on moments when you feel like you've lost control or are reacting automatically. These might be times when a protector part has taken over.

1. **Feeling Overwhelmed by Control**:
    - When have you felt completely controlled by a part?

- Example: "I felt overwhelmed when my perfectionist part took over, and I couldn't relax."
- My protector part took over when: _____

2. **Feeling Reactively Numb or Distracted:**
    - When do you feel like you've completely checked out or numbed yourself?
    - Example: "I felt like I couldn't stop binge-watching TV after a hard day."
    - My protector part took over when: _____

Step 2: Understanding Why Protectors Take Over

- **Instructions**: Reflect on the reasons behind your protector parts taking control.

1. What was your protector part trying to prevent or avoid?
    - Reflection: _____
2. What deeper emotions or exiles were being triggered at that moment?
    - Reflection: _____

Step 3: Regaining Balance

- **Instructions**: When protectors take over, the goal is to bring your Self back into the leadership role. Reflect on how you can invite your Self to take the lead when protectors become dominant.

1. How can you approach your protector parts with calmness and curiosity to regain balance?
    - Reflection: _____

2. What can you do to remind your protector that it doesn't have to carry all the weight?

    o Reflection: _____

Soothing Protectors

Worksheet 16: Offering Compassion to Protectors

Goal: To guide the user in offering compassion and understanding to their protector parts, acknowledging their efforts to keep the system safe.

Step 1: Acknowledging the Role of Your Protectors

- **Instructions**: Reflect on a specific protector part (manager or firefighter) that often steps in to keep you safe. Write down how this part has tried to protect you.

1. Which protector part are you reflecting on?

    o Example: "My critical part that pushes me to work harder."

    o My protector part is: _____

2. How has this part tried to keep you safe or prevent pain?

    o Reflection: _____

Step 2: Offering Compassion to the Protector

- **Instructions**: Write down something compassionate you can say to this protector part to acknowledge its efforts.

- Example: "I know you're working hard to protect me, and I appreciate everything you do to keep me safe."

Step 3: Inviting the Protector to Trust Your Self

- **Instructions**: Now, invite the protector part to trust your Self. Let it know that you are capable of leading and that it can rest.

1. What can you say to this part to reassure it that your Self is in charge?
    - Example: "I understand why you've been protecting me, and I'm here now to help take care of us."

Worksheet 17: Unburdening Protector Parts

Goal: To help the user release the burdens carried by their protector parts and allow these parts to take on healthier roles.

Step 1: Understanding the Burdens Carried by Protectors

- **Instructions**: Protector parts often carry heavy burdens, such as fear, guilt, or responsibility. Reflect on the burdens that your protector part may be carrying.

1. What burden does your protector part carry (e.g., fear, guilt, responsibility)?
    - Example: "My manager part carries the burden of perfectionism and fear of failure."
    - The burden my protector part carries is: _____

Step 2: Inviting the Protector to Release Its Burdens

- **Instructions**: Imagine having a conversation with your protector part, inviting it to release the burdens it has been carrying. What would it feel like to let go of these heavy burdens?

1. What can you say to your protector part to help it release its burdens?
    - Example: "You've been holding onto this fear for a long time, but it's okay to let go now."

Step 3: Visualizing the Unburdening

- **Instructions**: Close your eyes and imagine your protector part letting go of its burdens. Visualize it feeling lighter, freer, and at peace.

1. How does it feel to imagine your protector part being unburdened?
    - Reflection: _____
2. What new role can this part take on now that it no longer carries its burdens?
    - Reflection: _____

Worksheet 18: Creating Safe Spaces for Protectors

Goal: To help the user create safe internal spaces where their protector parts can feel supported and cared for, allowing them to rest.

Step 1: Visualizing a Safe Space

- **Instructions**: Close your eyes and imagine a peaceful, safe space where your protector part can rest. This could be a cozy room, a peaceful beach, or any place that feels comforting.

1. What does your safe space look like?

- Reflection: _____

2. How does your protector part feel in this space?

    - Reflection: _____

Step 2: Inviting Your Protector to Rest

- **Instructions**: Imagine inviting your protector part into this safe space. Let it know that it is safe and that it can rest here without needing to protect you constantly.

1. What can you say to your protector part to encourage it to rest?

    - Example: "You don't have to work so hard right now. It's safe for you to rest in this peaceful place."

Step 3: Checking in with Your Protector

- **Instructions**: Over time, check in with your protector part in its safe space. Ask it how it feels and whether it needs anything to feel comfortable.

1. What does your protector part need to feel more comfortable in its safe space?

    - Reflection: _____

Part 4: Healing Exiled Parts

These worksheets are designed to guide users through the process of connecting with and healing their exiled parts. By offering compassion, unburdening exiles, and creating safe relationships within their internal system, users can foster a deeper sense of emotional balance and well-being.

Connecting with Exiles

Worksheet 19: Recognizing Exiled Emotions

Goal: To help the user recognize the emotions that are held by their exiled parts, which have been suppressed or hidden to avoid emotional pain.

Step 1: Understanding Exiled Emotions

- **Instructions**: Read the following explanation.

Exiled parts are the parts of you that carry painful emotions, such as sadness, shame, fear, or guilt. These emotions are often too overwhelming to face, so your system pushes them aside to protect you. However, healing requires acknowledging and attending to these emotions with compassion.

Step 2: Identifying Exiled Emotions

- **Instructions**: Reflect on moments when you feel overwhelmed by certain emotions. These emotions might be linked to your exiles. Write down the feelings you often avoid or push away.

1. **Sadness**:
    - When do you feel deep sadness that you try to avoid?
    - Example: "I feel sad when I think about feeling alone or rejected."
    - My exiled sadness shows up when: _____

2. **Shame**:
    - When do you feel shame or unworthiness?

- Example: "I feel ashamed when I remember moments of failure."
- My exiled shame shows up when: _____

3. **Fear**:
   - When do you feel fearful or anxious, but push it away?
   - Example: "I avoid feeling fear by staying overly busy."
   - My exiled fear shows up when: _____

Step 3: Reflecting on Exiled Emotions

- **Instructions**: Reflect on how avoiding these emotions has affected your well-being.

1. What happens when you avoid or suppress these exiled emotions?
   - Reflection: _____
2. How do you think acknowledging these emotions could help you heal?
   - Reflection: _____

Step 4: Acknowledging Exiled Emotions with Compassion

- **Instructions**: Write down a compassionate statement that you can say to yourself as you begin to acknowledge your exiled emotions.
- Example: "I see your sadness, and I am here to hold space for you as you heal."

Worksheet 20: Exploring Childhood Exiles

Goal: To help the user explore exiled parts that carry painful emotions from childhood, allowing them to recognize and address early emotional wounds.

Step 1: Identifying Childhood Exiles

- **Instructions**: Think about experiences or emotions from your childhood that were too painful to deal with at the time. These emotions may have been exiled and are still carried by younger parts of you.

1. **Early Rejection or Loneliness**:
    - What childhood memories bring up feelings of rejection or loneliness?
    - Example: "I felt lonely when I was excluded from groups at school."
    - My childhood exile holds the memory of: _____

2. **Early Fear or Insecurity**:
    - What childhood experiences caused fear or insecurity?
    - Example: "I was afraid of being left out or unloved by my parents."
    - My childhood exile holds the memory of: _____

Step 2: Exploring the Emotions of Childhood Exiles

- **Instructions**: Reflect on the emotions your childhood exiles hold. What feelings were too overwhelming to face as a child, and how are they still present today?

1. What emotions did you suppress as a child that still feel unresolved?
    - Reflection: _____

2. How do these emotions influence your life today?

- Reflection: _____

Step 3: Offering Compassion to Your Childhood Exiles

- **Instructions**: Write down a compassionate message that you can offer to your childhood exiles.

- **Example**: "I see the fear and loneliness you felt as a child, and I am here to support you now."

Worksheet 21: Visualizing Exiles Safely
Goal: To help the user connect with their exiles in a safe and controlled way, using visualization to prevent overwhelm.

Step 1: Creating a Safe Space for Visualization

- **Instructions**: Before connecting with your exiled parts, it's important to create a safe space in your mind. Close your eyes and visualize a peaceful, protective space where your exiles can come forward.

1. What does this safe space look like?
    - Example: "A calm beach with gentle waves and warm sunshine."
    - My safe space looks like: _____

2. How do you feel in this space?
    - Reflection: _____

Step 2: Inviting Your Exile to Appear

- **Instructions**: Imagine gently inviting one of your exiled parts to come forward into your safe space. Let this part know it is safe here and that you are ready to listen.

1. Which exile are you inviting forward?
   - Example: "My exiled part that feels abandoned and afraid."
   - The exile I am inviting forward is:
     _____

2. What does this exile look or feel like as it appears in your visualization?
   - Reflection: _____

Step 3: Offering Reassurance and Support

- **Instructions**: As you visualize your exile, offer it reassurance and compassion. Let it know that it is safe to express its feelings.

1. What can you say to reassure your exile in this safe space?
   - Reflection: _____

Healing Process

Worksheet 22: Unburdening Exiled Parts

Goal: To help the user unburden their exiled parts by releasing the emotional pain and burdens these parts have been carrying.

Step 1: Understanding the Burdens of Your Exile

- **Instructions**: Reflect on the emotional burdens your exiled part is carrying. These might be feelings of shame, fear, guilt, or grief.

1. What emotional burdens does your exile carry?
   - Example: "My exile carries the burden of feeling unlovable."

- The burden my exile carries is:
  _____

Step 2: Inviting Your Exile to Release Its Burdens

- **Instructions**: Imagine having a conversation with your exile, inviting it to release its burdens. Let it know that it no longer has to carry this pain.

1. What can you say to help your exile release its burden?
   - Example: "You don't have to carry this pain anymore. You are safe now, and I am here for you."
2. How does your exile respond to this invitation to release its burdens?
   - Reflection: _____

Step 3: Visualizing the Unburdening

- **Instructions**: Close your eyes and visualize your exile letting go of its burdens. You might imagine the burdens being lifted away or transformed into lightness.

1. What does the unburdening process look like in your visualization?
   - Reflection: _____
2. How does your exile feel after releasing its burdens?
   - Reflection: _____

Worksheet 23: Offering the Self's Compassion to Exiles

Goal: To help the user offer their Self's compassion and healing presence to their exiled parts, supporting their exiles in feeling seen, heard, and cared for.

Step 1: Connecting with Your Self

- **Instructions**: Before offering compassion to your exile, take a few deep breaths and connect with your Self—the calm, compassionate core of who you are. Visualize your Self stepping forward with kindness and understanding.

1. How does it feel to connect with your Self?
    - Reflection: _____

Step 2: Offering Compassion to Your Exile

- **Instructions**: Imagine your Self sitting with your exile, offering it warmth and compassion. Gently acknowledge the pain your exile has been carrying.

1. What can you say to offer compassion to your exile?
    - Example: "I see your pain, and I am here to care for you."
    - My compassionate message to my exile is: _____

Step 3: Reassuring Your Exile

- **Instructions**: Reassure your exile that it is safe to feel its emotions and that it is no longer alone in its pain.

1. What can you say to let your exile know that it is safe now?
    - Reflection: _____
2. How does your exile respond to your Self's compassion?
    - Reflection: _____

Worksheet 24: Creating Safe Relationships Between Parts

Goal: To help the user foster safe, healthy relationships between their parts, allowing for harmony and balance within their internal system.

Step 1: Recognizing Conflict Between Parts

- **Instructions**: Reflect on any conflicts or tensions between your parts. These might be disagreements between protector parts and exiled parts or between manager and firefighter parts.

1. Which parts seem to be in conflict with one another?
    - Example: "My critical manager part and my exiled part that feels unworthy."
    - The parts in conflict are: _____
2. What emotions or concerns are causing this conflict?
    - Reflection: _____

Step 2: Inviting Your Self to Mediate

- **Instructions**: Imagine your Self stepping in to mediate between these parts, offering calmness and compassion to each. Encourage each part to express its feelings and needs.

1. What can you say to each part to help them feel heard and understood?
    - Reflection: _____
2. How does each part respond to your Self's presence?
    - Reflection: _____

Step 3: Creating Safe Relationships

- **Instructions**: Reflect on how you can create a safer, more harmonious relationship between these parts. This might involve reassuring protector parts that it's safe to let go, or helping exiled parts feel supported.

1. What steps can you take to foster a healthier relationship between your parts?
    - Reflection: _____
2. How can your Self continue to support these parts in building trust and safety?
    - Reflection: _____

Part 5: Integrating the Self

These worksheets in Part 5: Integrating the Self help users connect with their Self, strengthen their Self-leadership, and foster healing relationships within their internal system. By practicing Self-led conversations, bringing calm to their system, and rebuilding trust, users can achieve greater harmony and well-being

Getting in Touch with the Self

Worksheet 25: Visualizing the Self

Goal: To help the user connect with their Self, the calm, compassionate center within, and visualize the Self as the leader of their internal system.

Step 1: Understanding the Self

- **Instructions**: Read the following description of the Self.

The Self is your core—calm, compassionate, and confident. It is not a part, but the true essence of who you are. In Internal Family Systems (IFS), the Self is the leader of your internal system, able to heal and guide your parts with kindness and understanding.

Step 2: Visualizing Your Self

- **Instructions**: Close your eyes and take several deep breaths. Imagine a time when you felt calm, confident, and in control of your emotions. Visualize this version of yourself—your Self—stepping forward to lead.

1. How does your Self look or feel in this visualization?
    - Reflection: _____

2. What qualities does your Self bring into this visualization?
    - Example: "Calmness, compassion, and confidence."
    - Reflection: _____

Step 3: Strengthening Your Connection to the Self

- **Instructions**: Spend a few moments focusing on the qualities of your Self. Let these qualities fill your mind and body, and allow yourself to fully connect with your Self.

1. How does it feel to connect with your Self?
    - Reflection: _____

2. What message does your Self have for you in this moment?
    - Reflection: _____

Step 4: Bringing the Self into Daily Life

- **Instructions**: Write down one way you can bring your Self into your daily life. How can you invite your Self to take the lead in stressful or emotional situations?

- **Example**: "I can take a moment to pause and breathe before reacting, allowing my Self to guide me."

- **Reflection**: _____

Worksheet 26: Self-Led Conversations with Parts

Goal: To guide the user through a compassionate dialogue with their parts, led by their Self, to foster healing and understanding.

Step 1: Preparing for a Self-Led Conversation

- **Instructions**: Choose one part you would like to talk to. This could be a protector, exile, or any part that feels dominant right now. Take a few deep breaths and visualize your Self—calm, curious, and compassionate—stepping forward to lead this conversation.

1. Which part are you choosing to talk to?
    - Example: "My anxious part that worries about the future."
    - The part I will talk to is: _____

Step 2: Beginning the Conversation

- **Instructions**: Imagine your Self sitting with this part. Begin the conversation by asking the part how it is feeling and what it needs. Respond to the part with curiosity and compassion.

1. **Part**: "I feel anxious and overwhelmed. I don't know how to handle everything."
   Self: "I hear that you are feeling anxious. What do you need from me right now?"

- Continue the conversation, allowing your part to express its thoughts and feelings.

Step 3: Reflecting on the Conversation

- **Instructions**: Reflect on what you learned during this conversation. How did your Self respond to your part, and what insights did you gain?

1. What did you learn about this part and its needs?
   - Reflection: _____

2. How did your Self support or reassure this part?
   - Reflection: _____

Step 4: Moving Forward

- **Instructions**: Write down one way your Self can continue to support this part moving forward.

- Example: "I will remind this part that it is not alone and that my Self is here to lead."

- Reflection: _____

Worksheet 27: Bringing Calm to Your System

Goal: To help the user bring a sense of calm and balance to their internal system, especially during moments of emotional distress.

Step 1: Recognizing Distress in Your System

- **Instructions**: Think about a time when your internal system felt overwhelmed or chaotic. What were the emotions and parts that were most active during that time?

1. When did your system last feel chaotic or overwhelmed?
    - Reflection: _____

2. Which parts were most active during this time?
    - Reflection: _____

Step 2: Inviting Calm into Your System

- **Instructions**: Close your eyes and take a few deep breaths. Imagine your Self stepping forward and bringing calm to your internal system. Visualize your parts feeling reassured by the presence of your Self.

1. What does it feel like to invite calm into your system?
    - Reflection: _____

2. How do your parts respond to the presence of your Self?
    - Reflection: _____

Step 3: Practicing Calm in Daily Life

- **Instructions**: Write down one practice you can use to bring calm to your system during stressful moments. This might involve deep breathing, visualization, or simply pausing to reconnect with your Self.

- Example: "I will pause and take three deep breaths whenever I feel overwhelmed, allowing my Self to guide me."
- Reflection: _____

Self-Leadership

Worksheet 28: Leading from the Self in Conflict Situations

Goal: To help the user practice leading from their Self during moments of conflict, both internally and in relationships with others.

Step 1: Identifying a Recent Conflict

- **Instructions**: Think about a recent conflict you experienced, either internally (between your parts) or externally (with another person). Write down the details of the conflict.

1. What was the conflict?
    - Example: "I had an argument with a friend about feeling unsupported."
    - The conflict I experienced was: _____

2. Which parts of you were involved in this conflict?
    - Reflection: _____

Step 2: Reflecting on the Role of Your Self

- **Instructions**: Reflect on how your Self could have approached this conflict. What qualities of the Self (calmness, compassion, curiosity) could have helped resolve the situation?

1. How could your Self have approached this conflict differently?
   - Reflection: _____
2. What can you do next time to lead from your Self during a conflict?
   - Reflection: _____

Step 3: Practicing Self-Leadership

- **Instructions**: Write down one strategy you can use to lead from your Self in future conflicts. This might involve pausing, listening to your parts, or responding with curiosity and compassion.
- Example: "I will take a deep breath and listen to my parts before reacting, allowing my Self to guide the conversation."
- Reflection: _____

Worksheet 29: Trusting the Self to Guide Parts

Goal: To help the user build trust in their Self as the leader of their internal system, allowing their parts to feel safe and supported.

Step 1: Reflecting on Trust

- **Instructions**: Reflect on how much trust your parts currently have in your Self. Do they feel supported and safe under the Self's leadership, or do they still feel the need to take control?

1. How much do your parts trust your Self right now?
   - Reflection: _____
2. Which parts feel hesitant to trust the Self, and why?
   - Reflection: _____

Step 2: Building Trust Between Your Parts and Your Self

- **Instructions**: Imagine your Self sitting with one part that feels hesitant to trust. Have a conversation with this part, reassuring it that your Self is capable of leading.

1. What can your Self say to this part to build trust?
   - Example: "I understand that you've been protecting me for a long time, but I'm here now to guide us safely."
   - Reflection: _____

2. How does this part respond to your Self's reassurance?
   - Reflection: _____

Step 3: Strengthening the Leadership of the Self

- **Instructions**: Write down one practice you can use to strengthen the leadership of your Self and build trust with your parts.
- Example: "I will check in with my parts daily and remind them that my Self is here to guide and support them."
- Reflection: _____

Worksheet 30: Rebuilding Internal Relationships

Goal: To guide the user in rebuilding relationships between their parts, with the Self acting as a mediator and leader.

Step 1: Identifying Relationships That Need Healing

- **Instructions**: Reflect on relationships between your parts that may need healing. These could be conflicts between protector and exile parts or misunderstandings between different parts.

1. Which parts are in conflict or need healing?
    - Example: "My critical manager part and my vulnerable exile part."
    - The parts that need healing are: _____

Step 2: Inviting Your Self to Mediate

- **Instructions**: Visualize your Self stepping in to mediate between these parts. Let each part express its feelings and concerns, and respond with curiosity and compassion.

1. What do each of these parts need from your Self?
    - Reflection: _____
2. How can your Self help these parts find common ground or understanding?
    - Reflection: _____

Step 3: Rebuilding Relationships Between Parts

- **Instructions**: Write down one way your Self can help rebuild relationships between these parts, fostering harmony and balance in your internal system.
- **Example**: "I will remind my critical part to be gentle with my exile, and I will reassure my exile that it is safe now."
- Reflection: _____

Part 6: Advanced IFS Techniques

These worksheets in Part 6: Advanced IFS Techniques guide users through deeper and more complex aspects of Internal Family Systems, helping them build cohesion within their internal families, unburden long-held emotional pain, and work through trauma in a safe and supportive way.

Working with Internal Families

Worksheet 31: Building Cohesion in Your Internal System

Goal: To help the user create a sense of unity and cooperation within their internal system, where all parts work together under the leadership of the Self.

Step 1: Understanding Cohesion

- **Instructions**: Read the following explanation.

Cohesion in your internal system means that your parts work together as a team, each with its unique role but all guided by the Self. It is a state where parts no longer conflict with each other, but instead, cooperate in ways that support your overall well-being.

Step 2: Identifying Key Parts in Your System

- **Instructions**: Think about the main parts in your internal system. These could be protectors, exiles, or any other parts that frequently show up. Write down these key parts and their roles.

1. **Key Parts and Roles**:
    - Example: "My perfectionist part helps me stay organized, while my exile part carries feelings of sadness from the past."
    - The key parts in my system are:
      _____

Step 3: Strengthening Collaboration Between Parts

- **Instructions**: Reflect on how these parts could collaborate more effectively. What would it look like for them to work together under the guidance of your Self?

1. How can your protector parts support your exiles instead of taking over?
   - Reflection: _____
2. What can your Self do to encourage collaboration between these parts?
   - Reflection: _____

Step 4: Moving Toward Cohesion

- **Instructions**: Write down one action your Self can take to strengthen cohesion in your internal system.
- Example: "I will remind my perfectionist part that it doesn't need to overwork to keep me safe, and I will ask it to allow space for my exile's healing."
- Reflection: _____

Worksheet 32: Developing Compassion for All Parts

Goal: To help the user cultivate compassion for each part of their internal system, recognizing the important roles these parts play and supporting their healing.

Step 1: Understanding the Importance of Compassion

- **Instructions**: Read the following explanation.

Compassion is a key element in healing through IFS. When you approach your parts with compassion, they feel understood, supported, and safe. Even the parts that cause distress, such as protectors or firefighters, need compassion, as they are working hard to protect you in their own way.

Step 2: Identifying Parts That Need Compassion

- **Instructions**: Think about a part in your system that you struggle to accept or understand. Write down how this part shows up and what it might need from you.

1. Which part do you struggle to accept, and why?
    - Example: "My angry part often lashes out, and I find it hard to accept its presence."
    - The part I struggle with is: _____

2. What do you think this part needs from you in terms of compassion?
    - Reflection: _____

Step 3: Offering Compassion to Each Part

- **Instructions**: Take a few moments to offer compassion to this part. Imagine your Self sitting with this part, offering it understanding and kindness.

1. What can your Self say to offer compassion to this part?
    - Example: "I understand that you feel angry because you are trying to protect me, and I appreciate your efforts."
    - My compassionate message to this part is: _____

Step 4: Extending Compassion to Other Parts

- **Instructions**: Write down one way you can offer compassion to each of your key parts moving forward.

- Example: "I will check in with my critical part and let it know that I value its effort to keep me safe, but that I am now strong enough to lead."

- Reflection: _____

Worksheet 33: Resolving Long-Standing Conflicts Between Parts

Goal: To guide the user in resolving long-standing conflicts between parts, helping them to move toward internal harmony.

Step 1: Identifying Long-Standing Conflicts

- **Instructions**: Think about a conflict that has persisted between parts of your system for a long time. These conflicts could involve protector parts working against exiles or two protector parts trying to achieve conflicting goals.

1. Which parts are in long-standing conflict, and what are they fighting over?
    - Example: "My perfectionist part and my exile part have been at odds for years—one pushing me to work harder, while the other feels overwhelmed."
    - The parts in conflict are: _____
2. What is the source of this conflict?
    - Reflection: _____

Step 2: Understanding the Needs of Each Part

- **Instructions**: Reflect on the underlying needs of each part involved in the conflict. What are they trying to achieve or protect, and how can these needs be addressed in a way that benefits both parts?

1. What does each part need to feel heard and safe?
    - Reflection: _____
2. How can your Self step in to meet these needs and mediate the conflict?
    - Reflection: _____

Step 3: Moving Toward Resolution

- **Instructions**: Write down one way your Self can help resolve this long-standing conflict and bring peace to your system.

- **Example**: "I will reassure my perfectionist part that it's okay to take breaks, and I will offer my exile part support so it doesn't feel overwhelmed."

- Reflection: _____

Unburdening Techniques

Worksheet 34: Step-by-Step Guide to Unburdening
Goal: To help the user guide their parts through the process of unburdening, allowing them to release the heavy emotional burdens they carry.

Step 1: Identifying a Part Ready to Unburden

- **Instructions**: Think of a part that feels ready to release its burdens. This could be a protector, exile, or any other part that has been holding onto pain, fear, or responsibility.

1. Which part is ready to unburden, and what burdens does it carry?

    - Example: "My exile part carries the burden of feeling unworthy and rejected."

    - The part that is ready to unburden is: _____

Step 2: Inviting the Part to Let Go

- **Instructions**: Imagine sitting with this part and inviting it to let go of its burdens. Gently reassure the part that it no longer has to carry these feelings.

1. What can your Self say to help this part release its burdens?
    - Example: "It's okay to let go of this pain. You don't have to carry it anymore."
    - My Self says: _____

Step 3: Visualizing the Unburdening Process

- **Instructions**: Close your eyes and visualize the part letting go of its burdens. You might imagine the burdens being lifted away or transformed into lightness.

1. How does your part feel as it releases its burdens?
    - Reflection: _____
2. What new role can this part take on after unburdening?
    - Reflection: _____

Worksheet 35: Visualizing Safe Spaces for Exiles

Goal: To help the user create a safe internal space where their exiled parts can feel secure and supported, allowing for deeper healing.

Step 1: Creating a Safe Space

- **Instructions**: Close your eyes and imagine a peaceful, comforting space where your exiled parts can come forward. This space should feel completely safe and protected.

1. What does your safe space look like?

- Example: "A warm, cozy room with soft lighting and comforting sounds."
- My safe space looks like: _____

Step 2: Inviting Your Exile Into the Safe Space

- **Instructions**: Gently invite one of your exiled parts into this space. Let it know that it is safe here and that it can relax.

1. Which exile are you inviting into the safe space, and how does it respond?
   - Reflection: _____
2. What can you say to reassure your exile in this safe space?
   - Reflection: _____

Step 3: Strengthening the Sense of Safety

- **Instructions**: Reflect on how you can continue to create a sense of safety for your exiles. Write down one practice you can use to maintain this safe space.
- Example: "I will visualize this space each time my exile feels overwhelmed and remind it that it is safe here."
- Reflection: _____

Worksheet 36: Techniques for Deep Trauma Work

Goal: To guide the user through advanced techniques for working with deep-seated trauma, allowing their parts to release the pain in a safe, supported way.

Step 1: Identifying Trauma-Related Parts

- **Instructions**: Reflect on parts of your system that are connected to deep-seated trauma. These parts might carry memories, emotions, or fears related to past traumatic events.

1. Which parts are holding trauma-related pain, and what emotions are connected to this trauma?

    o   Reflection: _____

Step 2: Creating Safety for Trauma Work

- **Instructions**: Before engaging in trauma work, it is essential to create a safe and supportive environment. What can you do to create emotional safety for yourself and your parts?

1. How can you create safety for yourself and your parts during trauma work?

    o   Reflection: _____

Step 3: Gradually Unburdening Trauma

- **Instructions**: Trauma unburdening is a gradual process. Reflect on how your Self can gently guide your parts through this process, allowing them to release trauma at a safe pace.

1. What steps can your Self take to guide your parts through trauma work?

    o   Reflection: _____

2. How can your Self support your parts in unburdening trauma-related emotions?

    o   Reflection: _____

Step 4: Ongoing Support

- **Instructions**: Trauma healing requires ongoing support. Write down one practice you can use to continue supporting your parts after trauma work.

- Example: "I will check in with my parts regularly to make sure they feel safe and supported as we continue this healing journey."
- Reflection: _____

Part 7: Relationship between IFS and Trauma

These worksheets in Part 7: Relationship between IFS and Trauma guide users through understanding how trauma affects their parts, working with trauma-related firefighters and exiles, and creating safety before and during the healing process. By unburdening trauma-related parts and offering support and reassurance, users can foster a sense of safety and move toward deeper healing.

IFS in Trauma Recovery

Worksheet 37: Understanding How Trauma Affects Parts

Goal: To help the user understand how trauma influences the behavior and roles of their parts, especially protectors and exiles.

Step 1: Recognizing Trauma's Impact on Your Parts

- **Instructions**: Trauma can cause parts to take on extreme roles, such as protectors working overtime to prevent re-experiencing pain or exiles being pushed deeper into hiding. Reflect on how your parts may have been affected by past traumatic experiences.

1. How has trauma affected the roles of your protector parts?
    - Example: "My manager part became more controlling to prevent anything from going wrong."
    - Reflection: _____
2. How has trauma influenced your exiled parts?
    - Example: "My exile holds deep feelings of fear and shame from past events."
    - Reflection: _____

Step 2: Exploring Trauma's Influence on Your Internal System

- **Instructions**: Reflect on how trauma impacts your overall internal system. What dynamics or conflicts have emerged between your parts as a result of trauma?

1. How do your protector and exile parts interact in response to trauma?
    - Reflection: _____

2. What internal conflicts have arisen because of the trauma your parts are holding?

    o   Reflection: _____

Step 3: Moving Toward Understanding and Healing

- **Instructions**: Write down one way you can approach your trauma-affected parts with understanding and compassion.

- Example: "I will acknowledge the extra burden my protector parts are carrying and offer them gratitude for their efforts."

- Reflection: _____

Worksheet 38: Identifying Trauma-Related Firefighters

Goal: To help the user identify firefighter parts that have taken on specific roles in response to trauma, using distraction, numbing, or avoidance behaviors to soothe intense emotional pain.

Step 1: Recognizing Trauma-Related Firefighter Behaviors

- **Instructions**: Firefighter parts often react to trauma by using numbing or avoidance to protect you from overwhelming emotions. Reflect on how your firefighter parts have developed in response to trauma.

1. What behaviors do your firefighter parts use to distract or numb you from trauma-related pain?

    o   Example: "I binge-watch TV or overeat to avoid dealing with painful memories."

    o   My firefighter part distracts me by: _____

2. When do these firefighter parts typically become active?
   - Example: "When I feel triggered by reminders of past trauma."
   - My firefighter part becomes active when: _____

Step 2: Understanding the Motivation Behind Firefighter Parts

- **Instructions**: Firefighter parts act out of a need to protect you from trauma-related pain. Reflect on what your firefighter parts are trying to achieve by using these distraction or numbing strategies.

1. What is your firefighter part trying to prevent you from feeling?
   - Reflection: _____

2. How might this firefighter part feel if it didn't have to protect you from trauma anymore?
   - Reflection: _____

Step 3: Building a Relationship with Your Firefighter Parts

- **Instructions**: Write down one way you can start building a compassionate relationship with your firefighter parts, acknowledging their efforts while inviting them to trust your Self.

- Example: "I will thank my firefighter part for trying to protect me, but reassure it that I am strong enough to handle my emotions."

- Reflection: _____

Worksheet 39: Exploring Trauma-Related Exiles

Goal: To help the user explore their exiled parts that carry trauma-related pain, shame, fear, or sadness, and begin the process of gently connecting with these vulnerable parts.

Step 1: Recognizing Trauma-Related Exiles

- **Instructions**: Trauma-related exiles carry the deepest emotional pain from past events. Reflect on the emotions and memories your exiles hold that are related to trauma.

1. What trauma-related emotions do your exiled parts carry?
    - Example: "My exile holds feelings of abandonment and fear from a childhood trauma."
    - My trauma-related exile holds: _____

2. What memories are associated with these exiled emotions?
    - Reflection: _____

Step 2: Gently Connecting with Trauma-Related Exiles

- **Instructions**: Trauma-related exiles often feel hidden or isolated. Gently invite one of your exiles to come forward. Let it know that it is safe and that you are here to listen.

1. What can you say to reassure your exile that it is safe to come forward?
    - Example: "I know you've been holding this pain for a long time, but I am here to support you now."
    - Reflection: _____

2. How does your exile respond to this invitation to connect?
    - Reflection: _____

Step 3: Supporting Trauma-Related Exiles with Compassion

- **Instructions**: Write down one way you can continue to offer compassion and support to your trauma-related exiles as you move toward healing.
- Example: "I will remind my exile that it is no longer alone in its pain, and I will stay with it as it heals."
- Reflection: _____

Healing from Trauma

Worksheet 40: Unburdening Trauma in Firefighter Parts
Goal: To guide the user in helping their firefighter parts release the heavy burdens of trauma they've been carrying and find healthier ways to cope.

Step 1: Understanding the Burden of Trauma on Firefighter Parts

- **Instructions**: Firefighter parts often carry the burden of trying to manage intense trauma-related emotions. Reflect on what burdens your firefighter parts have been carrying in their efforts to protect you.

1. What burdens have your firefighter parts taken on due to trauma?
    - Example: "My firefighter part has taken on the burden of numbing me to prevent overwhelming emotions."
    - The burden my firefighter part carries is: _____

Step 2: Inviting Your Firefighter Parts to Release Their Burdens

- **Instructions**: Imagine having a conversation with your firefighter parts, inviting them to release their burdens. Let them know that they don't have to carry these burdens anymore.

1. What can you say to help your firefighter parts let go of their trauma-related burdens?

    - Example: "You don't need to numb the pain anymore. I am here to support us."
    - Reflection: _____

2. How does your firefighter part respond to this invitation to release its burdens?

    - Reflection: _____

Step 3: Moving Toward Healthier Coping Strategies

- **Instructions**: Write down one healthier way your firefighter part can cope with trauma-related emotions, with the support of your Self.
- Example: "Instead of avoiding the pain, I will take time to reflect and journal about my feelings when they come up."
- Reflection: _____

Worksheet 41: Supporting Exiles with Trauma

Goal: To help the user provide ongoing support and compassion to their exiled parts that carry trauma-related pain, offering them a path toward healing.

Step 1: Identifying the Needs of Trauma-Related Exiles

- **Instructions**: Trauma-related exiles often feel overwhelmed, abandoned, or fearful. Reflect on what these parts need from you to feel supported and safe.

1. What does your trauma-related exile need to feel safe and supported?

- Example: "My exile needs reassurance that it won't be abandoned again."
- Reflection: _____

Step 2: Offering Support and Reassurance

- **Instructions**: Imagine your Self sitting with your trauma-related exile, offering it kindness and reassurance. Write down what you can say to help this part feel safe.

1. What can your Self say to offer reassurance to your exile?
    - Example: "I see your pain, and I will stay with you. You are not alone anymore."
    - Reflection: _____

Step 3: Providing Ongoing Support

- **Instructions**: Write down one practice you can use to provide ongoing support to your trauma-related exiles, ensuring that they feel safe throughout the healing process.
- Example: "I will check in with my exile daily and remind it that I am here for as long as it needs me."
- Reflection: _____

Worksheet 42: Creating Safety Before Healing Trauma

Goal: To help the user create a safe internal environment for trauma healing, ensuring that their parts feel supported before engaging in deeper trauma work.

Step 1: Understanding the Importance of Safety

- **Instructions**: Before healing trauma, it is essential to create emotional safety for your parts. Reflect on what safety looks like for your system and how you can create this supportive environment.

1. What does emotional safety look like for your parts?
    - Example: "My parts need to know that they won't be overwhelmed by painful emotions."
    - Reflection: _____

Step 2: Creating a Safe Environment for Trauma Work

- **Instructions**: Write down one way you can create a safe environment for your parts before starting trauma healing. This might involve grounding exercises, visualization, or taking breaks when needed.

1. What can you do to ensure your parts feel safe before engaging in trauma work?
    - Reflection: _____

Step 3: Inviting Your Parts to Trust the Process

- **Instructions**: Let your parts know that they can trust the healing process and that you will be there to guide them safely. Reassure them that they can take the process at their own pace and that their feelings will be respected.

1. What can your Self say to reassure your parts that it is safe to begin trauma healing?
    - Example: "We will go slow, and I won't let anything overwhelm us. You are safe with me."
    - Reflection: _____

Step 4: Maintaining Safety Throughout the Healing Process

- **Instructions**: Write down one practice you can use to ensure that your parts continue to feel safe throughout the trauma healing process. This might include regular check-ins, grounding exercises, or creating a comforting ritual.

1. How will you maintain a sense of safety during trauma work?
    - Example: "I will take breaks during deep trauma work and check in with my parts to make sure they feel supported."
    - Reflection: _____

Part 8: Practical Applications of IFS

These worksheets in Part 8: Practical Applications of IFS guide users through applying IFS in various life situations, including work, relationships, and conflict. Each worksheet encourages ongoing Self-leadership and offers space for therapist feedback to reinforce progress and reflection.

IFS in Daily Life

Worksheet 43: Applying IFS at Work

Goal: To help the user apply IFS principles in their work environment, using the Self to lead and manage parts that may become activated during work-related stress or challenges.

Step 1: Recognizing Work-Related Parts

- **Instructions**: Reflect on which parts become active during your workday. These may be parts that push you to succeed, avoid conflict, or protect you from failure.

1. Which parts show up the most at work, and what are their roles?
    - Example: "My perfectionist part pushes me to work extra hard, while my avoidant part tries to steer me away from difficult tasks."
    - My work-related parts are: _____

Step 2: Identifying Triggers at Work

- **Instructions**: Think about situations at work that trigger specific parts. Write down how these triggers affect your parts and the overall dynamic at work.

1. What triggers activate your parts at work, and how do they respond?
    - Example: "When I'm assigned a new project, my perfectionist part takes over and demands extra effort."
    - My triggers at work are: _____

Step 3: Applying Self-Leadership in Work Situations

- **Instructions**: Reflect on how your Self can step in to lead your work-related parts, offering calm, compassionate guidance.

1. How can your Self guide these parts to manage work challenges more effectively?
    - Example: "My Self can remind my perfectionist part that doing my best is enough and that I don't need to overwork."
    - Reflection: _____

Therapist Comments/Feedback:

- "Great awareness of how your parts show up at work. Continue practicing Self-leadership, especially in high-stress moments, to balance your perfectionist part and avoid burnout."

Worksheet 44: Using IFS in Relationships

Goal: To guide the user in applying IFS principles in relationships, helping them understand how parts show up in relational dynamics and how the Self can lead to healthier connections.

Step 1: Recognizing Parts in Relationships

- **Instructions**: Reflect on the parts that become active in your relationships, especially during moments of conflict or emotional intensity.

1. Which parts tend to show up in your close relationships, and what roles do they play?
    - Example: "My caretaker part always wants to make others happy, while my critical part gets activated when I feel unappreciated."

- My relational parts are: _____

Step 2: Identifying Relationship Triggers

- **Instructions**: Think about specific situations in relationships that activate your parts. Write down how these triggers affect your interactions with others.

1. What triggers your parts in relationships, and how do they respond?
    - Example: "When my partner is distant, my caretaker part becomes anxious and overextends itself."
    - My relationship triggers are: _____

Step 3: Using the Self to Lead in Relationships

- **Instructions**: Reflect on how your Self can guide your parts to maintain healthy boundaries and compassion in relationships.

1. How can your Self help balance your parts in relationships, especially during conflicts?
    - Example: "My Self can remind my caretaker part that it's okay to set boundaries and that I don't have to solve every problem."
    - Reflection: _____

Therapist Comments/Feedback:

- "Good insight into how your caretaker part shows up. Keep practicing boundaries, allowing your Self to lead interactions with compassion for both yourself and others."

Worksheet 45: Parts Activation in Conflict Situations

Goal: To help the user recognize which parts become activated during conflicts and guide their Self to take the lead in resolving these situations.

Step 1: Identifying Parts in Conflict

- **Instructions**: Think about a recent conflict you experienced. Reflect on which parts were activated during that conflict.

1. Which parts were most active during the conflict, and how did they behave?
    - Example: "My defensive part took over and made me shut down, while my critic part judged the other person."
    - My conflict-related parts are:
    _____

Step 2: Recognizing Triggers in Conflict

- **Instructions**: Reflect on what triggered the conflict and how it affected your parts. Write down how your parts responded to these triggers.

1. What was the trigger that set off the conflict, and how did your parts react?
    - Example: "The conflict started when my colleague questioned my work, and my defensive part immediately shut down communication."
    - The conflict trigger was: _____

Step 3: Guiding Parts with the Self During Conflict

- **Instructions**: Reflect on how your Self can step in to guide your parts during conflicts, helping to resolve issues with clarity and calmness.

1. How can your Self lead your parts through conflict resolution?
   - Example: "My Self can help my defensive part stay open to communication, instead of shutting down."
   - Reflection: _____

Therapist Comments/Feedback:
- "Great job identifying how your defensive part operates. With more practice, your Self can take the lead earlier in conflicts, helping you remain open and communicative."

Maintaining Self-Leadership

Worksheet 46: Recognizing When Parts Take Over
Goal: To help the user recognize when parts take over and how to regain Self-leadership during challenging moments.

Step 1: Identifying When Parts Take Over
- **Instructions**: Reflect on a time when a part took over and led you away from your calm, centered Self.

1. Describe a recent moment when a part took control. Which part was it, and how did it behave?
   - Example: "My anxious part took over when I was preparing for a big presentation, making me feel overwhelmed."
   - The part that took over was: _____

Step 2: Reflecting on the Impact of Parts Taking Over

- **Instructions**: Write down how this part's actions affected you and what the consequences were.

1. How did this part's takeover affect your actions and emotions?
   - Reflection: _____

Step 3: Bringing the Self Back to Lead

- **Instructions**: Reflect on how your Self can step in to regain leadership when a part takes over. What can you do to bring calmness back?

1. How can your Self guide you back to balance when a part takes over?
   - Example: "I can pause, take a deep breath, and ask my anxious part to step back so I can lead."
   - Reflection: _____

Therapist Comments/Feedback:

- "It's great that you noticed when your anxious part took over. Pausing and taking a breath is an excellent way to invite your Self back into the lead."

Worksheet 47: Returning to the Self in Challenging Situations

Goal: To guide the user in returning to Self-leadership during challenging or emotionally intense situations, allowing them to respond with calmness and compassion.

Step 1: Recognizing When You've Lost Self-Leadership

- **Instructions**: Reflect on a challenging situation where you felt disconnected from your Self. What was happening at the time, and which part took over?

1. Describe the situation where you lost connection with your Self.
    - Example: "During a family argument, I felt my defensive part take control, and I lost my sense of calm."
    - The situation was: _____

Step 2: Using the Self to Regain Balance

- **Instructions**: Think about how you could reconnect with your Self during a challenging situation. What practices can help you regain balance?

1. What can you do to reconnect with your Self in challenging moments?
    - Example: "I can take a break, breathe deeply, and remind myself that I am capable of handling the situation with compassion."
    - Reflection: _____

Step 3: Practicing Self-Leadership in Difficult Moments

- **Instructions**: Write down one way you can practice Self-leadership during a future challenging situation.
- **Example**: "Next time I feel defensive in a conversation, I will pause and speak from a place of curiosity instead of reacting defensively."
- Reflection: _____

Therapist Comments/Feedback:

- "Excellent work reflecting on how to return to your Self during challenges. Keep practicing, and this process will become more natural over time."

Worksheet 48: Daily Practices to Maintain Self-Leadership

Goal: To help the user develop daily practices that keep them connected to their Self, allowing them to maintain balance and calm leadership throughout their day.

Step 1: Reflecting on Your Daily Routine

- **Instructions**: Think about your daily routine. What moments throughout the day tend to activate your parts and make you lose connection with your Self?

1. When do you tend to lose Self-leadership during your daily routine?
    - Example: "I often lose connection with my Self when I'm rushing to meet deadlines."
    - Reflection: _____

Step 2: Developing Daily Self-Leadership Practices

- **Instructions**: Reflect on what daily practices you can introduce to stay connected with your Self. This might include mindfulness, meditation, journaling, or taking mindful breaks.

1. What practices can you include in your daily routine to maintain Self-leadership?
    - Example: "I will practice a five-minute meditation in the morning to start my day with calmness."
    - Reflection: _____

Step 3: Committing to Daily Self-Leadership

- **Instructions**: Write down one specific Self-leadership practice you will commit to doing daily, and reflect on how it will benefit you.

1. What is your daily Self-leadership practice, and how will it help you stay balanced?
    - Example: "I will journal for 10 minutes at the end of each day to reflect on how my parts showed up and how I stayed connected to my Self."
    - Reflection: _____

Therapist Comments/Feedback:

- "This is a wonderful daily practice! Staying mindful of how your parts show up each day will help you maintain Self-leadership consistently."

Part 9: Specialized Worksheets for Creative Expression

These worksheets in **Part 9: Specialized Worksheets for Creative Expression** provide creative outlets for users to explore and heal their parts through art, writing, and visualization. The creative approaches offer a unique way to deepen the connection between parts and the Self, fostering emotional release and healing. Each worksheet concludes with a space for therapist feedback, reinforcing the user's growth and insights.

Creative Approaches to IFS

Worksheet 49: Using Art to Express Parts

Goal: To help the user express their internal parts visually, using creative art as a way to connect with and understand their parts.

Step 1: Choosing a Part to Express Through Art

- **Instructions**: Reflect on one of your internal parts that you'd like to explore. This could be a protector, exile, or any part that feels present. Choose a part that you are ready to express through art.

1. Which part are you choosing to express through art?
    - Example: "I'm choosing my perfectionist part, which always wants me to do everything perfectly."
    - The part I am expressing is: _____

Step 2: Creating Art to Express Your Part

- **Instructions**: Use any medium (drawing, painting, collage, etc.) to express this part visually. Let go of any judgment and allow your creative expression to reflect the feelings, qualities, or characteristics of this part.

1. What did you create, and how does it reflect your part's role, feelings, or behavior?
    - Example: "I drew a figure that's holding a long list of tasks, symbolizing my perfectionist part's need to control everything."
    - My artwork represents: _____

Step 3: Reflecting on Your Creative Expression

- **Instructions**: Reflect on the artwork you've created. How does it help you understand this part better?

1. How does your artwork reveal new insights about this part's motivations or feelings?
    - Reflection: _____

Therapist Comments/Feedback:

- "This is a beautiful exploration of your part through art. Continue using creative expression as a way to bring deeper understanding to the emotions and needs of your parts."

Worksheet 50: Writing Dialogues Between Parts

Goal: To guide the user in writing dialogues between their parts, allowing them to explore conflicts, needs, and resolutions through creative writing.

Step 1: Choosing Parts for Dialogue

- **Instructions**: Choose two parts that often interact with or conflict with each other. These could be protector parts, exiles, or any combination of parts that you feel need a conversation.

1. Which two parts are you choosing to dialogue with each other?
    - Example: "I'm choosing my anxious part and my nurturing part."
    - The two parts I'm working with are: _____

Step 2: Writing the Dialogue

- **Instructions**: Write a dialogue between these two parts, allowing each part to express its feelings, needs, and concerns. Let the conversation flow naturally, without judgment or editing.

1. **Anxious Part**: "I'm worried that something will go wrong. We have to prepare for the worst."
   Nurturing Part: "I hear that you're anxious, but it's okay to take a break. I'll take care of things for now."

- Continue the dialogue, letting the parts express themselves freely.

Step 3: Reflecting on the Dialogue

- **Instructions**: Reflect on what you learned from this dialogue between your parts. What insights or resolutions emerged?

1. What new understanding did you gain from the dialogue between your parts?
   - Reflection: _____

2. How can your Self support these parts moving forward?
   - Reflection: _____

Therapist Comments/Feedback:

- "This written dialogue reveals important dynamics between your parts. Keep exploring these conversations to deepen your understanding of their relationship."

Worksheet 51: Expressing Burdens Through Creativity

Goal: To help the user express the burdens their parts carry using a creative medium, allowing for a deeper understanding of the emotional weight these burdens hold.

Step 1: Identifying a Burden to Express

- **Instructions**: Reflect on a burden that one of your parts is carrying. This could be a feeling of guilt, fear, shame, or any emotional weight that your part holds. Choose a creative medium (art, writing, music, etc.) to express this burden.

1. Which burden are you choosing to express, and which part carries this burden?
    - Example: "My exile part carries the burden of feeling unworthy."
    - The burden I am expressing is: _____

Step 2: Expressing the Burden Creatively

- **Instructions**: Use your chosen medium to express the burden your part carries. Focus on conveying the emotional weight of this burden through your creative process.

1. What did you create, and how does it represent the burden?
    - Example: "I wrote a poem about feeling lost and unseen, which reflects my exile's burden of unworthiness."
    - My creation represents: _____

Step 3: Reflecting on Your Creative Expression

- **Instructions**: Reflect on how this creative expression helped you connect with the burden your part carries. What insights or emotions emerged during this process?

1. What did you learn about the burden your part is carrying?
    - Reflection: _____

Therapist Comments/Feedback:

- "This is a powerful way to express your part's burden. Creative outlets like this can be incredibly healing. Keep using these methods to explore and release emotional weight."

Creative Healing

Worksheet 52: Visualizing the Healing Process

Goal: To help the user visualize the healing process for one of their parts, using imagery and creative visualization to support the release of emotional burdens.

Step 1: Visualizing the Healing of a Part

- **Instructions**: Choose one part that you feel is ready for healing. Close your eyes and visualize this part going through the healing process. Imagine it releasing its burdens and feeling lighter, supported, and free.

1. Which part are you visualizing, and what burdens is it releasing?
    - Example: "I'm visualizing my anxious part, releasing its fear of failure."
    - The part I am visualizing is: _____

Step 2: Creating a Visual Representation of Healing

- **Instructions**: Create a visual representation of your part's healing process. This could be a drawing, painting, or any other visual medium that helps you capture the feeling of healing and release.

1. What did you create, and how does it represent your part's healing journey?
    - Reflection: _____

Step 3: Reflecting on the Healing Process

- **Instructions**: Reflect on how visualizing the healing process helped you connect with your part's journey. What emotions or insights emerged during this process?

1. How did this visualization support your part's healing?
    - Reflection: _____

Therapist Comments/Feedback:

- "Your visualization of healing is a powerful tool. It's important to keep nurturing this process, allowing your parts to experience relief and transformation through creative visualization."

Worksheet 53: Creating a Safe Haven for Exiles Through Art

Goal: To guide the user in creating a safe haven for their exiled parts using art, providing these vulnerable parts with a space where they feel protected and supported.

Step 1: Visualizing a Safe Haven for Your Exile

- **Instructions**: Close your eyes and imagine a safe, comforting place where your exiled part can feel completely secure. Visualize this space in as much detail as possible, focusing on how it feels to be there.

1. Describe the safe haven you visualized for your exile.

- Example: "I imagined a cozy forest cabin with soft lighting and a warm fire, where my exile feels safe."
- My safe haven looks like: _____

Step 2: Creating Your Safe Haven Through Art

- **Instructions**: Use any art medium to create your safe haven. Focus on expressing the feeling of safety and security that this space provides for your exile.

1. What did you create, and how does it represent safety for your exile?
   - Reflection: _____

Step 3: Reflecting on the Safe Haven

- **Instructions**: Reflect on how this artistic representation of a safe haven can help your exile feel protected. How does your exile respond to being in this space?

1. How does your exile feel in this safe haven?
   - Reflection: _____

Therapist Comments/Feedback:

- "This safe haven is a beautiful gift for your exile. Keep using it as a retreat for your vulnerable parts whenever they need comfort or protection."

Worksheet 54: Journaling as a Form of Healing

Goal: To help the user use journaling as a way to process emotions, connect with their parts, and support the healing process.

Step 1: Choosing a Part to Journal With

- **Instructions**: Choose one part that you would like to focus on during this journaling session. This could be a part that is currently active or one that is seeking attention.

1. Which part are you choosing to journal with, and why?
    - Example: "I'm choosing to journal with my inner critic, who often makes me feel inadequate."
    - The part I'm journaling with is: _____

Step 2: Writing from the Part's Perspective

- **Instructions**: Write from the perspective of this part. Let it express its feelings, thoughts, and needs in an uncensored way. Allow the part to speak freely through your writing.

What did your part express through journaling?

- Example: "My inner critic expressed frustration about wanting me to succeed and feeling disappointed when I don't meet expectations."
- My part expressed: _____

Step 3: Reflecting on the Journal Entry

- **Instructions**: Reflect on what you learned from this journaling session. How did it help you understand your part better, and what insights did you gain about its needs?

1. What new insights did you gain about this part?
    - Reflection: _____
2. How can your Self support this part moving forward?
    - Reflection: _____

Therapist Comments/Feedback:

- "Journaling can be a powerful tool for self-discovery. You're gaining important insights about your inner critic's motivations. Keep journaling with your parts to continue building this relationship."

Part 10: Reflection and Growth

These worksheets in **Part 10: Reflection and Growth** guide users through reflecting on their IFS journey, tracking their progress, and setting goals for future growth. Each worksheet encourages users to deepen their connection with their Self, while the therapist comments and tips offer ongoing support and reinforcement of these practices.

Reflecting on Your IFS Journey

Worksheet 55: Reflecting on Progress in Healing Parts

Goal: To guide the user in reflecting on the progress they have made in healing their parts and understanding how their relationship with their parts has evolved.

Step 1: Identifying Healing Progress

- **Instructions**: Think about one or more parts that have undergone significant healing during your IFS journey. Reflect on how these parts have changed and how your relationship with them has evolved.

1. Which parts have experienced healing, and how have they changed?
   - Example: "My anxious part is less reactive, and I'm more able to reassure it when it becomes activated."
   - The parts that have healed are: _____

2. How has your relationship with these parts shifted?
   - Reflection: _____

Step 2: Acknowledging Your Role in Healing

- **Instructions**: Reflect on how your Self has played a role in this healing process. How have you led with compassion, curiosity, and calmness to support your parts?

1. How has your Self supported these parts in their healing?
   - Reflection: _____

Step 3: Celebrating Healing Milestones

- **Instructions**: Write down one specific milestone in your healing journey that you are proud of.

1. What is a healing milestone you've achieved, and how has it impacted your overall well-being?
    - Reflection: _____

Tips:

- Take time to acknowledge even small steps in healing. Every bit of progress is meaningful.
- Healing is not linear—parts may fluctuate in how they feel over time, and that's okay.

Therapist Comments/Feedback:

- "It's wonderful to see the progress you've made in healing your parts. Keep celebrating these milestones, and remember that healing is an ongoing process."

Worksheet 56: Journaling Your Growth in Self-Leadership

Goal: To help the user reflect on their growth in leading their internal system with the Self and how this has influenced their interactions with their parts and the world.

Step 1: Recognizing Self-Led Growth

- **Instructions**: Think about how your ability to lead with your Self has grown over time. Reflect on specific moments where you noticed your Self leading your internal system with calmness and compassion.

1. In what ways have you noticed growth in your Self-leadership?
    - Example: "I've become better at pausing during stressful situations and responding with calm instead of reacting impulsively."
    - My Self-led growth looks like: _____

Step 2: Noticing External Changes

- **Instructions**: Reflect on how this growth in Self-leadership has affected your interactions with others and how you handle external challenges.

1. How has your increased Self-leadership changed how you interact with others or manage external stress?
    - Reflection: _____

Step 3: Journaling Your Progress

- **Instructions**: Take a few minutes to journal about a recent experience where you led with your Self, focusing on how it felt and how it impacted the outcome.

1. Describe a recent experience where your Self took the lead. How did it feel, and what was the outcome?
    - Reflection: _____

Tips:

- Keep a journal to track moments where your Self takes the lead—it helps reinforce Self-leadership.
- Recognize that even small shifts in leading with your Self make a big difference over time.

Therapist Comments/Feedback:

- "It's great to see your growing ability to lead with your Self. Journaling these experiences will help you stay connected to this progress."

Worksheet 57: Understanding Changes in Your Internal System

Goal: To help the user reflect on the changes they've noticed in their internal system as parts begin to heal, communicate, and find balance under the leadership of the Self.

Step 1: Noticing Shifts in Your Parts

- **Instructions**: Reflect on the changes you've noticed in the way your parts interact with each other and how your internal system has shifted over time.

1. How has your internal system changed since beginning your IFS journey?
    - Example: "My protector parts are less rigid, and my exiles feel safer coming forward."
    - The changes in my system are: _____

Step 2: Reflecting on System Dynamics

- **Instructions**: Think about how these shifts have affected the dynamics between your parts. Are conflicts less frequent? Are your parts working together more harmoniously?

1. How have the dynamics between your parts changed, and what new patterns have emerged?
    - Reflection: _____

Step 3: Acknowledging Positive System Changes

- **Instructions**: Write down one specific change in your internal system that you feel has been most impactful to your emotional well-being.

1. What is the most impactful change you've noticed in your internal system, and how has it helped you?
    - Reflection: _____

Tips:

- Regularly check in with your internal system to notice and appreciate subtle changes.
- Balance takes time—be patient with your parts as they adjust to new dynamics.

Therapist Comments/Feedback:

- "Your system is becoming more balanced and connected, which is a huge achievement. Keep checking in with your parts regularly to nurture this progress."

Future Growth

Worksheet 58: Setting Goals for Continued Healing

Goal: To help the user set realistic and meaningful goals for continued healing and growth within their IFS journey.

Step 1: Reflecting on Future Healing Goals

- **Instructions**: Think about the areas where you would like to continue healing. These could be specific parts that need more attention, or broader areas like emotional resilience, boundaries, or self-compassion.

1. What are your goals for continued healing?
    - Example: "I want to work on building more trust with my exiled parts and feel more comfortable expressing emotions."
    - My healing goals are: _____

Step 2: Breaking Down Your Goals

- **Instructions**: Break down your healing goals into smaller, actionable steps that you can work on over time.

1. What are the smaller steps you can take to achieve these goals?
    - Reflection: _____

Step 3: Committing to Growth

- **Instructions**: Write down one commitment you will make to continue your healing journey.

1. What is one commitment you are making to support your healing growth?
    - Reflection: _____

Tips:

- Set realistic goals that feel achievable, and celebrate small victories along the way.
- Check in with your healing goals periodically and adjust them as needed.

Therapist Comments/Feedback:

- "You've set meaningful goals for continued healing. Breaking them into smaller steps will help you stay on track. Be patient with yourself and acknowledge every bit of progress."

Worksheet 59: Building a Supportive Internal System

Goal: To help the user build a supportive internal system where parts work together under the Self's leadership, fostering a sense of safety and cooperation.

Step 1: Recognizing Supportive Parts

- **Instructions**: Identify parts of your internal system that are naturally supportive and helpful in your daily life. These might be parts that help with organization, self-care, or emotional regulation.

1. Which parts are most supportive, and how do they help you in your daily life?
    - Example: "My nurturing part helps me practice self-compassion when I'm feeling down."
    - My supportive parts are: _____

Step 2: Fostering Collaboration Between Parts

- **Instructions**: Reflect on how you can encourage more collaboration between your parts, especially between protector and exile parts. What would it look like for your parts to work together more effectively?

1. How can you foster more collaboration between your parts?
    - Reflection: _____

Step 3: Building a Stronger Internal Support System

- **Instructions**: Write down one specific action you can take to strengthen the sense of support within your internal system.

1. What is one thing you can do to build a more supportive internal system?
    - Reflection: _____

Tips:

- Encourage dialogue between your parts regularly to keep your internal system cohesive.
- Remember that each part plays an important role—acknowledge and appreciate their efforts.

Therapist Comments/Feedback:

- "Your internal system is becoming more cohesive. Continue fostering these relationships, and your parts will feel even more supported by your Self."

Worksheet 60: Creating Daily Self-Led Practices
Goal: To help the user create daily practices that reinforce Self-leadership, ensuring that their internal system remains balanced and supported.

Step 1: Identifying Daily Self-Led Practices

- **Instructions**: Think about what practices you can incorporate into your daily routine to keep your Self at the forefront of your internal system. This could include mindfulness, meditation, journaling, or any activity that helps you stay grounded.

1. What daily practices will help you maintain Self-leadership?

- Example: "I will start each day with a five-minute mindfulness meditation to connect with my Self."
- My daily Self-led practices are: _____

Step 2: Committing to Your Practices

- **Instructions**: Write down your commitment to practicing these Self-led activities daily, and reflect on how these practices will benefit your internal system over time.

1. What benefits do you expect from consistently practicing Self-leadership?
   - Example: "I expect to feel more balanced and calm, even during stressful situations, and my parts will trust my Self more."
   - Reflection: _____

Step 3: Adapting Practices as Needed

- **Instructions**: Reflect on how you will adapt your practices if challenges arise or if certain activities feel less effective over time.

1. How can you adjust your daily Self-led practices to fit your changing needs?
   - Example: "If I feel overwhelmed, I can shorten my meditation or practice journaling instead."
   - Reflection: _____

Tips:

- Consistency is key. Even small daily practices can have a profound effect on your system over time.

- Be flexible with your practices—adjust them as needed to fit your emotional state or schedule.

Therapist Comments/Feedback:

- "Creating daily practices to maintain Self-leadership is a wonderful way to stay grounded. Consistency will strengthen your connection to your Self, and adapting these practices as needed will keep them relevant and effective."

Part 11: Tracking Emotions and Triggers

These worksheets in Part 11: Tracking Emotions and Triggers guide users through daily reflections on their emotions and triggers, as well as monthly reviews of their healing journey. By staying aware of emotional patterns, shifts in parts, and progress in unburdening, users can track their growth and set clear intentions for future healing. Each worksheet includes tips and therapist feedback to reinforce ongoing self-awareness and growth.

Daily Reflection Worksheets

Worksheet 61: Identifying Emotions of the Day

Goal: To help the user track and reflect on the emotions they experienced throughout the day, gaining awareness of patterns and triggers.

Step 1: Identifying Your Emotions

- **Instructions**: Reflect on the main emotions you felt throughout the day. Write down how each emotion manifested and in which situations it was most intense.

1. What were the dominant emotions you experienced today, and what situations triggered these emotions?
    - Example: "I felt anxious during a meeting, and later I felt relief after finishing a project."
    - The emotions I experienced today are: _____

Step 2: Reflecting on Emotional Intensity

- **Instructions**: Rate the intensity of each emotion on a scale from 1 to 10, with 10 being the most intense.

1. How intense were these emotions throughout the day?
    - Example: "My anxiety during the meeting was an 8, but my relief afterward was a 4."
    - Emotion intensity ratings: _____

Step 3: Noticing Patterns

- **Instructions**: Reflect on any patterns you noticed in your emotions. Were certain emotions linked to specific times of the day, people, or situations?

1. Did you notice any patterns in your emotions today?
    - Reflection: _____

Tips:

- Tracking your emotions regularly helps build emotional awareness and identify triggers.
- Use this worksheet to recognize how your emotions fluctuate during different times of the day or in specific contexts.

Therapist Comments/Feedback:

- "Great job reflecting on your emotions. Keep tracking these feelings daily to build more awareness of how your emotions shift throughout the day."

Worksheet 62: Trigger Response Worksheet

Goal: To guide the user in recognizing triggers that activate emotional responses and understanding how their parts respond to these triggers.

Step 1: Identifying the Trigger

- **Instructions**: Reflect on a situation that triggered an emotional response today. Write down what the trigger was and what emotion or reaction it activated.

1. What was the trigger, and how did you respond emotionally or behaviorally?

- Example: "The trigger was a colleague criticizing my work, and it made me feel defensive and anxious."
- The trigger today was: _____

Step 2: Recognizing Which Parts Were Activated

- **Instructions**: Reflect on which parts of you were activated in response to the trigger. What role did these parts play in protecting you or responding to the situation?

1. Which parts were activated by this trigger, and how did they respond?
    - Example: "My defensive part took over, trying to shield me from feeling hurt."
    - The parts that were activated are:
      _____

Step 3: Exploring Alternative Responses

- **Instructions**: Reflect on how your Self could lead differently if faced with the same trigger in the future. What can you do to stay connected to your Self when triggered?

1. How can your Self lead you differently next time this trigger arises?
    - Reflection: _____

Tips:

- Triggers can be opportunities for growth. By reflecting on them, you can gain better control over your emotional reactions.
- Use this worksheet to identify which parts are most vulnerable to specific triggers and how to respond more effectively.

Therapist Comments/Feedback:

- "You're doing a great job identifying your triggers and parts. Continue reflecting on these moments to build more resilience and stay connected to your Self."

Worksheet 63: Checking in with Parts

Goal: To help the user check in with their parts at the end of the day, fostering communication and understanding within their internal system.

Step 1: Identifying Active Parts

- **Instructions**: Reflect on which parts were most active today. Write down how they showed up and what role they played in your daily experiences.

1. Which parts were most present today, and how did they influence your thoughts, feelings, or actions?
    - Example: "My manager part was very present during work, helping me stay on track with my tasks."
    - The active parts today were: _____

Step 2: Listening to Your Parts' Needs

- **Instructions**: Take a moment to listen to your parts. What do these parts need from you right now? Do they need rest, reassurance, or acknowledgment?

1. What do your active parts need from you today?
    - Reflection: _____

Step 3: Offering Compassion to Your Parts

- **Instructions**: Write down a compassionate statement you can offer to one of your active parts, showing appreciation for its role.

1. How can you show compassion and gratitude to one of your parts today?
    - Example: "I appreciate my manager part for helping me stay organized, and I'll allow it to rest now."
    - Reflection: _____

Tips:

- Regular check-ins with your parts help foster internal harmony and balance.
- Acknowledge the efforts of your parts, even those that may cause discomfort. They are all trying to help in their own way.

Therapist Comments/Feedback:

- "This check-in process is a wonderful way to build a deeper connection with your parts. Keep offering them compassion and listening to their needs."

Tracking Progress Over Time

Worksheet 64: Monthly Review of Healing

Goal: To help the user review their progress in healing over the past month, reflecting on changes in their internal system and emotional well-being.

Step 1: Reflecting on Healing Progress

- **Instructions**: Look back over the past month. Which parts have experienced the most healing, and how have your emotions shifted?
1. Which parts have healed the most, and how has this healing changed your emotional landscape?
    - Example: "My anxious part has softened, and I'm feeling more at peace overall."
    - My healing progress this month is: _____

Step 2: Noticing Changes in Emotional Resilience

- **Instructions**: Reflect on how your emotional resilience has changed. Are you better able to handle stress, triggers, or emotional challenges?
1. How has your emotional resilience improved over the past month?
    - Reflection: _____

Step 3: Setting Intentions for Next Month

- **Instructions**: Write down one goal or intention you have for your healing journey in the upcoming month.
1. What is one healing goal you have for the next month?
    - Reflection: _____

Tips:

- Take time to reflect each month on how far you've come. Healing is an ongoing journey.
- Celebrate your progress, no matter how small. Each step forward matters.

Therapist Comments/Feedback:

- "You've made incredible progress this month. Keep setting small goals and reflecting on your growth—it will motivate you to continue your healing journey."

Worksheet 65: Assessing Shifts in Parts and Self-Leadership

Goal: To guide the user in assessing the shifts they've noticed in their parts and their Self-leadership over time.

Step 1: Noticing Shifts in Parts

- **Instructions**: Reflect on how your parts have changed over time. Have certain parts become less reactive or more cooperative?

1. How have your parts shifted in their roles, reactions, or interactions?
    - Example: "My critical part has become less judgmental, and my protector parts are allowing me to lead more often."
    - The shifts I've noticed in my parts are: _____

Step 2: Assessing Self-Leadership Growth

- **Instructions**: Reflect on how your ability to lead with your Self has evolved. Are you more capable of guiding your parts with compassion and calmness?

1. How has your Self-leadership grown, and how has this impacted your internal system?
    - Reflection: _____

Step 3: Setting Future Intentions for Self-Leadership

- **Instructions**: Write down one intention for continuing to strengthen your Self-leadership moving forward.

1. What is one intention you have for strengthening Self-leadership?
   - Reflection: _____

Tips:

- Regularly assess how your parts are evolving, as well as how your Self is growing.
- Trust the process—shifts in parts and Self-leadership take time, but each step brings you closer to balance.

Therapist Comments/Feedback:

- "It's great to see the positive shifts in your parts and Self-leadership. Continue focusing on these changes as you move forward in your healing journey."

Worksheet 66: Healing and Unburdening Journey Tracker

Goal: To help the user track their progress in healing and unburdening parts over time, offering a clear overview of their journey.

Step 1: Tracking Healing Milestones

- **Instructions**: Write down the key milestones in your healing and unburdening journey so far. Which parts have been unburdened, and what has been their transformation?

1. What healing milestones have you achieved, and how have your parts transformed?

- Example: "My protector part has let go of its fear of failure and now supports me in staying calm."
- My healing milestones are: _____

Step 2: Reflecting on the Impact of Unburdening

- **Instructions**:

Reflect on the impact that unburdening has had on your overall emotional well-being and internal system. How have you felt since these parts released their burdens?

1. How has unburdening your parts impacted your emotional well-being and internal balance?
   - Example: "Since unburdening my critical part, I feel less pressure to be perfect, and I'm more at peace with myself."
   - The impact of unburdening has been: _____

Step 3: Setting Future Unburdening Goals

- **Instructions**: Think about any parts that are still carrying burdens. Write down one or more goals you have for future unburdening and healing work with these parts.

1. What unburdening goals do you have for the future, and which parts need attention?
   - Reflection: _____

Tips:

- Tracking your progress helps reinforce the importance of healing and motivates you to continue.

- Be patient with yourself—unburdening is a gradual process, and each step forward is significant.

Therapist Comments/Feedback:

- "You've made remarkable progress in your unburdening journey. Keep setting goals for the parts that still need healing, and celebrate the transformations that have already taken place."

Part 12: Addressing Specific Client Issues

These worksheets in **Part 12: Addressing Specific Client Issues** help users navigate complex emotional experiences like anxiety, depression, trauma, shame, and addiction. Each worksheet includes tips for practical application and therapist feedback to reinforce growth, healing, and self-compassion.

Working with Anxiety

Worksheet 67: Identifying Parts Triggered by Anxiety

Goal: To help the user identify which parts are triggered by anxiety and how they manifest in different situations.

Step 1: Identifying the Parts

- **Instructions**: Reflect on the moments when you feel anxious. Identify which parts are triggered by anxiety and how they respond.

1. Which parts are most often triggered by anxiety, and what are their reactions?
    - Example: "My perfectionist part gets triggered and makes me feel like I need to control everything."
    - The parts triggered by anxiety are: _____

Step 2: Recognizing Anxiety-Driven Behaviors

- **Instructions**: Write down how these parts influence your behavior when you are feeling anxious.

1. How do these anxious parts affect your actions and decisions?
    - Reflection: _____

Step 3: Noticing Patterns in Anxiety

- **Instructions**: Reflect on the patterns you've noticed in how anxiety-triggered parts show up in specific situations.

1. What patterns have you noticed about when and how your anxiety parts become active?

- Reflection: _____

Tips:

- Start by tracking how anxiety affects you during daily activities, and look for repeating triggers.
- Keep a journal to help identify which parts are involved in your anxiety and their specific roles.

Therapist Comments/Feedback:

- "Great work identifying the parts involved in your anxiety. Keep noticing patterns, and soon you'll see how each part tries to help in its own way."

Worksheet 68: Soothing Anxious Parts Through Self-Compassion

Goal: To guide the user in offering self-compassion to the parts that experience anxiety, creating a sense of safety and support.

Step 1: Identifying Anxious Parts

- **Instructions**: Reflect on a specific anxious part that you would like to focus on in this exercise.

1. Which anxious part are you focusing on, and what is its main concern?
    - Example: "My worried part is always anxious about the future."
    - The part I am focusing on is: _____

Step 2: Offering Compassion to the Anxious Part

- **Instructions**: Imagine your Self sitting with this anxious part. Offer it compassion by acknowledging its worries and reassuring it with kindness.

1. What compassionate statement can you say to this part?
    - Example: "I know you're worried about what might happen, but we're going to be okay. I'm here for you."
    - Reflection: _____

Step 3: Reflecting on the Soothing Process

- **Instructions**: Reflect on how offering compassion affected your anxious part.

1. How did your part respond to the compassion and reassurance you offered?
    - Reflection: _____

Tips:

- Regularly offering compassion to your anxious parts can reduce the intensity of their worries.
- Practice deep breathing or mindfulness before offering compassion to help ground yourself.

Therapist Comments/Feedback:

- "Your effort to offer compassion to your anxious parts is a powerful step. Keep practicing, and over time, these parts will feel more reassured by your Self's presence."

Worksheet 69: Recognizing the Role of Firefighters in Anxiety Management

Goal: To help the user recognize how firefighter parts respond to anxiety by using distraction, numbing, or avoidance behaviors to manage overwhelming emotions.

Step 1: Identifying Firefighter Behaviors

- **Instructions**: Reflect on how your firefighter parts respond when you feel anxious. Do they use distraction, avoidance, or other behaviors to manage your anxiety?

1. What behaviors do your firefighter parts engage in to cope with anxiety?
    - Example: "My firefighter part makes me zone out on social media when I feel anxious."
    - My firefighter parts manage anxiety by: _____

Step 2: Understanding the Motivation Behind Firefighters

- **Instructions**: Reflect on why your firefighter parts use these behaviors. What are they trying to protect you from?

1. What are your firefighter parts trying to prevent you from feeling?
    - Reflection: _____

Step 3: Reflecting on the Impact of Firefighter Behaviors

- **Instructions**: Write down how these firefighter behaviors affect your ability to process anxiety.

1. How do firefighter behaviors help or hinder your ability to cope with anxiety?

- Reflection: _____

Tips:

- Firefighters often have good intentions, but their methods may lead to avoidance rather than resolution.
- Recognizing these patterns helps you understand how to work with your firefighter parts.

Therapist Comments/Feedback:

- "It's insightful to recognize how your firefighter parts manage anxiety. With practice, you can support these parts in finding healthier ways to cope."

Worksheet 70: Developing Self-Leadership to Manage Anxiety

Goal: To help the user practice Self-leadership in managing anxiety, guiding their anxious parts with calmness and confidence.

Step 1: Reflecting on Self-Leadership During Anxiety

- **Instructions**: Think of a time when your Self was able to manage an anxious situation. Reflect on how you stayed connected to your Self during that moment.

1. How did your Self handle anxiety in this situation?
    - Example: "I stayed calm and reminded myself that I was capable of handling the problem."
    - Reflection: _____

Step 2: Using Self-Leadership to Reassure Anxious Parts

- **Instructions**: Imagine your Self stepping in to guide your anxious parts. What can you say to these parts to reassure them and maintain calm?

1. How can your Self lead your anxious parts through future situations?
    - Reflection: _____

Step 3: Developing a Self-Led Anxiety Response Plan

- **Instructions**: Write down a plan for how your Self will respond to anxiety in the future. Include steps to stay grounded and reassure your anxious parts.

1. What is your Self-led plan for managing anxiety?
    - Reflection: _____

Tips:

- Practice Self-leadership in small anxiety-provoking situations to build confidence.
- Use grounding techniques like deep breathing or mindfulness to stay connected to your Self during anxious moments.

Therapist Comments/Feedback:

- "Your ability to stay connected to your Self during anxious moments is key to managing anxiety. Keep practicing, and you'll feel more empowered over time."

Working with Depression

Worksheet 71: Identifying Exiled Parts Connected to Depression

Goal: To help the user identify exiled parts that are connected to feelings of depression and how these parts influence their emotional state.

Step 1: Identifying Depression-Related Exiles

- **Instructions**: Reflect on your feelings of depression and which exiled parts might be holding these emotions. These could be parts carrying sadness, hopelessness, or shame.

1. Which exiled parts do you think are connected to your depression?
    - Example: "My exile part carries the burden of feeling unworthy."
    - The exiled parts connected to my depression are: _____

Step 2: Understanding the Emotions of Exiled Parts

- **Instructions**: Write down the emotions these exiled parts are holding and how they influence your overall emotional state.

1. What emotions are your exiled parts holding, and how do they affect you?
    - Reflection: _____

Step 3: Offering Support to Exiled Parts

- **Instructions**: Reflect on how you can offer support and compassion to these exiled parts, acknowledging their pain.

1. What can you do to help your exiled parts feel seen and supported?
    - Reflection: _____

Tips:

- Depression-related exiles often feel isolated. Offering them acknowledgment is the first step toward healing.
- Take small steps in reconnecting with these parts, as they may be deeply burdened.

Therapist Comments/Feedback:

- "Your awareness of the exiled parts connected to your depression is powerful. Continue offering them support, and you'll begin to feel lighter."

Worksheet 72: Exploring the Burden of Hopelessness

Goal: To help the user explore feelings of hopelessness carried by their exiled parts and understand how these burdens impact their emotional state.

Step 1: Recognizing Hopelessness in Exiled Parts

- **Instructions**: Reflect on moments when you feel hopeless or stuck. Identify which parts carry these feelings of hopelessness.

1. Which exiled parts are holding the burden of hopelessness, and when do they become active?
    - Example: "My exiled part that feels abandoned carries the belief that nothing will ever get better."
    - The exiled parts carrying hopelessness are: _____

Step 2: Understanding the Impact of Hopelessness

- **Instructions**: Write down how these feelings of hopelessness influence your daily life, emotions, and energy levels.

1. How does hopelessness affect your actions, emotions, and outlook on life?
    - Reflection: _____

Step 3: Offering Compassion to Hopeless Parts

- **Instructions**: Reflect on what your hopeless parts need to feel supported and seen. Write down a compassionate message you can offer to these parts.

1. What compassionate statement can you offer to your hopeless parts?
    - Example: "I see how heavy this burden is, and I'm here to support you as we move through this together."
    - Reflection: _____

Tips:

- Hopelessness often emerges from a place of deep pain. Offering small moments of hope and acknowledgment can be healing.
- Be patient—hopeless parts may take time to trust that change is possible.

Therapist Comments/Feedback:

- "Your willingness to connect with the hopeless parts of yourself shows great courage. Keep offering compassion, and over time, these parts will begin to feel supported."

Worksheet 73: Understanding the Role of Protector Parts in Depression

Goal: To help the user understand how protector parts may contribute to or manage feelings of depression and how these parts attempt to shield exiles from emotional pain.

Step 1: Identifying Depression-Related Protector Parts

- **Instructions**: Reflect on which protector parts are trying to manage or control feelings of depression. These parts may try to numb emotions or avoid triggers.

1. Which protector parts are involved in managing your depression, and how do they behave?
    - Example: "My avoidant part keeps me from facing painful feelings, making me feel disconnected."
    - The protector parts connected to my depression are: _____

Step 2: Recognizing the Intentions of Protector Parts

- **Instructions**: Reflect on what these protector parts are trying to achieve. Are they trying to shield you from pain, prevent you from feeling too much, or manage other emotions?

1. What are these protector parts trying to accomplish, and why do they use these strategies?
    - Reflection: _____

Step 3: Offering Support to Protectors

- **Instructions**: Write down how you can offer your protector parts reassurance that they no longer need to carry this burden alone.

1. What can you say to your protector parts to help them trust that your Self can handle the situation?

    - Reflection: _____

Tips:

- Protectors often use behaviors like avoidance or numbing to manage depression. Recognizing this can help you work with them.
- Acknowledge the efforts of your protector parts while gently reassuring them that you are ready to take the lead.

Therapist Comments/Feedback:

- "Your insight into the role of protector parts in depression is valuable. Keep building trust with these parts, letting them know that they don't have to carry the load alone."

Worksheet 74: Offering Compassion to Exiled Parts with Depression

Goal: To guide the user in offering compassion and support to exiled parts carrying depression, helping these parts feel seen and understood.

Step 1: Connecting with Depressed Exiles

- **Instructions**: Reflect on a specific exiled part that is carrying depression. Take a moment to sit with this part and acknowledge its pain.

1. Which exiled part are you focusing on, and what feelings of depression is it holding?

    - Example: "My exiled part feels sadness and loss from a difficult childhood experience."

- The part I'm focusing on is: _____

Step 2: Offering Compassion to the Depressed Part

- **Instructions**: Imagine your Self sitting with this exiled part. Offer it words of compassion, acknowledging its struggles and pain.

1. What compassionate message can you offer to this exiled part?
    - Example: "I see the sadness you've been carrying, and I'm here to listen and support you."
    - Reflection: _____

Step 3: Reflecting on the Process

- **Instructions**: Write down how your exiled part responded to your compassionate presence and what you learned from this process.

1. How did your exiled part respond to the compassion you offered?
    - Reflection: _____

Tips:

- Compassion is a powerful tool in healing depression-related exiles. Offering a kind and non-judgmental presence can create a sense of safety.
- Take small steps in connecting with these parts, as they may be carrying significant emotional weight.

Therapist Comments/Feedback:

- "Your ability to offer compassion to your exiled parts is a crucial step in healing. Keep practicing this gentle approach, and over time, these parts will begin to trust your Self more."

Working with Trauma

Worksheet 75: Mapping Trauma-Related Parts

Goal: To help the user map the parts of their internal system that are connected to trauma, identifying how these parts respond to or carry the effects of trauma.

Step 1: Identifying Trauma-Related Parts

- **Instructions**: Reflect on how trauma has impacted your internal system. Identify the parts that are directly connected to trauma—whether as exiles carrying pain or protectors managing the trauma.

1. Which parts of your system are most affected by trauma, and how do they manifest?
    - Example: "My firefighter part tries to avoid trauma reminders by distracting me, while my exile part holds the sadness."
    - The trauma-related parts in my system are: _____

Step 2: Mapping the Interactions Between Parts

- **Instructions**: Reflect on how these trauma-related parts interact with each other. Are they in conflict? Do protectors prevent exiles from expressing themselves?

1. How do your trauma-related parts interact with each other?
    - Reflection: _____

Step 3: Understanding the Trauma-Driven Dynamics

- **Instructions**: Write down any patterns you notice about how trauma affects your internal system as a whole.

1. What patterns have you observed in how trauma influences your system's dynamics?
    - Reflection: _____

Tips:

- Mapping out your trauma-related parts can help you see the bigger picture of how trauma affects your internal system.
- Take time with this process, as trauma-related parts often carry heavy burdens and may be slow to reveal themselves fully.

Therapist Comments/Feedback:

- "This is excellent work identifying and mapping your trauma-related parts. Keep exploring these dynamics, and you'll start to see how healing is possible."

Worksheet 76: Building Safety Before Addressing Trauma

Goal: To help the user create emotional and psychological safety before engaging in trauma work, ensuring that they feel grounded and supported.

Step 1: Establishing a Safe Space

- **Instructions**: Before working with trauma-related parts, it's important to create a sense of safety. Close your eyes and imagine a peaceful, protected space where your parts can feel safe.

1. What does your safe space look like, and how does it make you feel?
    - Reflection: _____

Step 2: Inviting Your Parts Into the Safe Space

- **Instructions**: Imagine inviting one of your trauma-related parts into this safe space. Let it know that it is safe here and that it doesn't have to face the trauma alone.

1. Which part are you inviting into the safe space, and how does it respond?
    - Reflection: _____

Step 3: Reflecting on the Safety Process

- **Instructions**: Reflect on how creating safety affects your ability to work with trauma-related parts.

1. How does this process of building safety support your healing journey?
    - Reflection: _____

Tips:

- Always prioritize safety when working with trauma. Trauma parts need to know they are safe before they can begin healing.
- Use grounding techniques, like deep breathing or visualization, to reinforce the sense of safety.

Therapist Comments/Feedback:

- "Building safety is essential when addressing trauma. You're doing a great job creating a safe environment for your parts, which will make deeper trauma work possible."

Worksheet 77: Unburdening Trauma-Related Exiles

Goal: To guide the user in the process of helping their trauma-related exiles release the emotional burdens they carry, facilitating healing and relief.

Step 1: Identifying the Trauma Burdens

- **Instructions**: Reflect on the specific burdens that your trauma-related exiled parts are holding. These burdens might include fear, shame, grief, or anger.

1. What emotional burdens are your trauma-related exiles carrying?
    - Example: "My exile is holding onto feelings of helplessness and fear from a traumatic event in childhood."
    - The burdens my exiled parts carry are: _____

Step 2: Inviting Your Exiles to Release Their Burdens

- **Instructions**: Imagine sitting with one of your trauma-related exiles and gently inviting it to let go of its burdens. Reassure the part that it no longer has to carry these heavy emotions alone.

1. What can your Self say to your exile to encourage it to release its burdens?
    - Example: "You don't have to hold onto this pain anymore. I'm here with you, and it's safe to let it go."
    - Reflection: _____

Step 3: Visualizing the Unburdening Process

- **Instructions**: Close your eyes and visualize your exile letting go of its burdens. Imagine these burdens being lifted away or transformed into lightness.

1. How did your exile respond to the invitation to release its burdens, and how do you feel after the process?

    - Reflection: _____

Tips:

- Be patient with trauma-related exiles—unburdening is often a gradual process that requires time and trust.
- Create a safe, calm environment when working with trauma-related parts to ensure they feel supported.

Therapist Comments/Feedback:

- "Your willingness to help your exiled parts release their burdens is a big step. Keep working slowly and gently with these parts, and they will feel safer to unburden over time."

Worksheet 78: Developing a Trauma-Sensitive Self-Leadership Approach

Goal: To help the user develop a compassionate, trauma-sensitive approach to Self-leadership that prioritizes safety, empathy, and understanding when working with trauma-related parts.

Step 1: Understanding Trauma-Sensitive Leadership

- **Instructions**: Reflect on what it means to lead your internal system in a trauma-sensitive way. This involves leading with patience, gentleness, and a deep sense of empathy for your trauma-related parts.

1. What does trauma-sensitive Self-leadership look like to you, and how can it benefit your healing journey?

- Example: "It means approaching my trauma parts with extra care and being patient with the healing process."
- Reflection: _____

Step 2: Leading with Compassion

- **Instructions**: Think about a time when your trauma-related parts needed compassion. How can you offer them the compassion and safety they need while maintaining Self-leadership?

1. How can you ensure that your trauma-related parts feel safe under your Self's leadership?
   - Reflection: _____

Step 3: Creating a Trauma-Sensitive Leadership Plan

- **Instructions**: Write down a plan for how you will lead your internal system through trauma work, ensuring that all parts feel supported and safe throughout the process.

1. What is your trauma-sensitive leadership plan, and how will it help you manage the healing process?
   - Reflection: _____

Tips:

- A trauma-sensitive approach requires extra patience and understanding. Make sure your parts know that they can take their time to heal.
- Use calming techniques like grounding or mindfulness before engaging with trauma-related parts to help maintain a trauma-sensitive mindset.

Therapist Comments/Feedback:

- "Your approach to leading with a trauma-sensitive perspective is insightful. Continue focusing on providing safety and compassion to your trauma-related parts, and healing will follow."

Working with Shame

Worksheet 79: Identifying Shame-Based Parts

Goal: To help the user identify parts that carry shame and understand how these parts influence feelings of worthlessness, guilt, or inadequacy.

Step 1: Identifying Shame-Based Parts

- **Instructions**: Reflect on which parts carry feelings of shame. These parts might carry beliefs such as "I'm not good enough," or "I'm unworthy."

1. Which parts in your internal system are holding onto shame, and how do they manifest?
    - Example: "My exiled part feels shame from being criticized as a child, and it makes me feel unworthy of love."
    - The shame-based parts in my system are: _____

Step 2: Recognizing Shame's Impact

- **Instructions**: Write down how these shame-based parts influence your self-esteem, relationships, or overall emotional state.

1. How do these parts and their shame affect your life and relationships?
    - Reflection: _____

Step 3: Connecting with Shame-Based Parts

- **Instructions**: Reflect on how you can offer support to these parts, helping them feel seen and understood without judgment.

1. How can you begin to connect with these shame-based parts in a compassionate way?
    - Reflection: _____

Tips:

- Shame-based parts often feel isolated. Offering acknowledgment and understanding is the first step toward healing.
- Remember, shame is often rooted in old experiences. Addressing it with kindness can bring relief to your parts.

Therapist Comments/Feedback:

- "Your ability to recognize shame-based parts is crucial to your healing process. Keep offering these parts compassion, and over time, they'll begin to release their burdens."

Worksheet 80: Understanding the Protective Role of Shame

Goal: To help the user understand that shame-based parts often serve a protective function, attempting to shield them from further emotional pain.

Step 1: Recognizing Shame as a Protector

- **Instructions**: Reflect on how your shame-based parts might be trying to protect you from feeling even more vulnerable or exposed.

1. How do you think your shame-based parts are protecting you from further emotional harm?

- - Example: "My shame-based part criticizes me so that I don't take risks and get hurt."
  - Reflection: _____

Step 2: Exploring the Intention Behind Shame

- **Instructions**: Write down what your shame-based parts are trying to achieve by making you feel small or inadequate.

1. What is your shame-based part's goal in making you feel shame?
   - Reflection: _____

Step 3: Reassuring Your Shame-Based Parts

- **Instructions**: Reflect on how you can reassure your shame-based parts that they don't need to protect you in this way anymore.

1. What can you say to your shame-based parts to help them feel safe and less burdened?
   - Reflection: _____

Tips:

- Shame-based parts often act as protectors to avoid deeper pain. Understanding this can help you approach them with compassion.
- Take time to explore the role of shame without judgment—it's likely trying to protect you in ways you might not have realized.

Therapist Comments/Feedback:

- "Understanding shame as a protective mechanism can shift how you approach it. Keep reassuring your shame-based parts, and they'll start to let go of their protective roles."

Worksheet 81: Healing Exiled Parts with Shame Burdens

Goal: To guide the user in healing exiled parts that carry the burden of shame by offering them compassion, understanding, and validation.

Step 1: Identifying the Burdens of Shame

- **Instructions**: Reflect on a specific exiled part that carries shame. Write down the nature of the shame it is carrying and how long it has been holding onto this burden.

1. What shame burden is this exiled part carrying, and what is the origin of this shame?

    - Example: "My exile feels ashamed about being rejected as a child, and it still carries that belief."
    - The shame burden my exile carries is: _____

Step 2: Offering Compassion to Shame-Based Exiles

- **Instructions**: Imagine your Self sitting with this shame-based exile, offering it compassion and understanding. Acknowledge its pain and let it know that it no longer has to carry this shame alone.

1. What compassionate statement can you offer to your exile to begin healing the shame?

    - Example: "You don't need to feel ashamed for being who you are. I see you, and I'm here for you."
    - Reflection: _____

Step 3: Reflecting on the Healing Process

- **Instructions**: Write down how your shame-based exile responded to your Self's compassion and how the healing process began to unfold.

1. How did your exile respond to the compassion you offered, and what shifts have you noticed?
   - Reflection: _____

Tips:

- Healing shame-based exiles can be a slow process. Be gentle with these parts, as they may have been carrying their burdens for a long time.
- Return to these exiles often to reinforce the message that they are worthy of love and acceptance.

Therapist Comments/Feedback:

- "Your compassion for your shame-based exiled parts is essential for healing. Keep showing them kindness, and they'll start to release the shame they've been holding onto."

Worksheet 82: Replacing Shame with Self-Compassion

Goal: To help the user replace the feelings of shame within their internal system with self-compassion, promoting self-acceptance and healing.

Step 1: Identifying Where Shame Shows Up

- **Instructions**: Reflect on where shame tends to show up most strongly in your life. This could be in certain situations, relationships, or in response to specific triggers.

1. In which areas of your life does shame show up most frequently, and how does it affect you?

- Example: "I feel shame when I make mistakes at work, and it makes me doubt my abilities."
- The situations where shame shows up are: _____

Step 2: Replacing Shame with Self-Compassion

- **Instructions**: Think of a recent situation where shame appeared. How can you respond to yourself with self-compassion instead of judgment or criticism?

1. How can you replace the feeling of shame with self-compassion in this situation?
   - Example: "Instead of criticizing myself for making a mistake, I will remind myself that everyone makes mistakes, and it's okay."
   - Reflection: _____

Step 3: Practicing Self-Compassion Daily

- **Instructions**: Write down one self-compassionate practice that you will incorporate into your daily routine to help replace shame with acceptance and kindness.

1. What is one daily practice you will use to show yourself more compassion?
   - Reflection: _____

Tips:

- Catch yourself in moments when shame arises and gently shift your inner dialogue to one of compassion.
- Self-compassion is a skill that grows with practice—start with small steps and build from there.

Therapist Comments/Feedback:
- "Your focus on replacing shame with self-compassion is a wonderful shift. Keep practicing this daily, and over time, you'll notice a significant change in how you relate to yourself."

Working with Addiction

Worksheet 83: Understanding Firefighter Parts and Addiction

Goal: To help the user understand the role of firefighter parts in addictive behaviors and how these parts use addiction as a way to manage overwhelming emotions.

Step 1: Recognizing Firefighter Parts

- **Instructions**: Reflect on which firefighter parts use addictive behaviors to cope with overwhelming emotions. Identify the situations where these parts become active.

1. Which firefighter parts engage in addictive behaviors, and what emotions are they trying to avoid or manage?
    - Example: "My firefighter part turns to alcohol to numb feelings of loneliness."
    - The firefighter parts connected to addiction are: _____

Step 2: Exploring the Role of Addiction

- **Instructions**: Write down how addiction serves as a coping mechanism for these parts. What are they trying to achieve by engaging in addictive behaviors?

1. How do these parts believe addiction is helping you manage emotional pain?
    - Reflection: _____

Step 3: Offering Alternatives to Firefighter Parts

- **Instructions**: Reflect on how you can offer your firefighter parts healthier alternatives to manage their emotions without resorting to addictive behaviors.

1. What healthier coping strategies can you offer your firefighter parts to help them manage emotions differently?
    - Reflection: _____

Tips:

- Recognizing the role of firefighter parts in addiction helps reframe addictive behaviors as attempts to manage emotional pain, not personal failure.
- Offering healthier coping strategies can help firefighter parts feel supported and reduce their reliance on addictive behaviors.

Therapist Comments/Feedback:

- "You're gaining valuable insight into how your firefighter parts use addiction as a coping mechanism. Keep exploring healthier alternatives, and over time, these parts will learn new ways to manage difficult emotions."

Worksheet 84: Mapping the Cycle of Addiction in Your Internal System

Goal: To help the user map how addiction cycles through their internal system, identifying triggers, firefighter behaviors, and the effects on their overall emotional state.

Step 1: Identifying the Addiction Cycle

- **Instructions**: Reflect on how the cycle of addiction moves through your internal system. Write down the triggers that activate firefighter parts and how the cycle unfolds.

1. What are the main triggers for your addictive behaviors, and how does the cycle of addiction progress?
    - Example: "When I feel stressed, my firefighter part urges me to escape through addictive behaviors, which leads to guilt afterward."
    - The addiction cycle in my system is: _____

Step 2: Recognizing the Impact of Addiction

- **Instructions**: Write down how the cycle of addiction affects your overall emotional well-being and how it impacts your internal parts.

1. How does the addiction cycle affect your parts and your emotional state?
    - Reflection: _____

Step 3: Breaking the Addiction Cycle

- **Instructions**: Reflect on how you can begin to break the addiction cycle by addressing triggers, offering healthier coping strategies, and supporting your firefighter parts.

1. What steps can you take to start breaking the addiction cycle?

- Reflection: _____

Tips:

- Mapping out the addiction cycle helps you understand the patterns that drive it, making it easier to disrupt and change.
- Focus on small, manageable steps to break the cycle, such as recognizing triggers early and responding with healthier behaviors.

Therapist Comments/Feedback:

- "You're doing important work by mapping out your addiction cycle. With time and practice, you can begin to shift these patterns and support your parts in healthier ways."

Worksheet 85: Building Compassion for Parts Engaging in Addictive Behaviors

Goal: To help the user build compassion for the parts that engage in addictive behaviors, recognizing that these parts are trying to help manage pain, even if their methods are harmful.

Step 1: Understanding the Motivation Behind Addictive Behaviors

- **Instructions**: Reflect on what your firefighter parts are trying to achieve through addictive behaviors. What emotional needs are they trying to meet?

1. What emotional needs are your firefighter parts trying to address through addiction?
    - Example: "My firefighter part is trying to help me feel calm and avoid stress."

- Reflection: _____

Step 2: Offering Compassion to Firefighter Parts

- **Instructions**: Imagine sitting with your firefighter parts and offering them compassion. Let them know you understand their struggles and that you want to help them find healthier ways to cope.

1. What can you say to your firefighter parts to show them compassion and understanding?
   - Reflection: _____

Step 3: Developing a Plan for Healthier Coping

- **Instructions**: Write down one or two healthier strategies you can offer to your firefighter parts as alternatives to addiction.

1. What healthier strategies will you use to support your firefighter parts in managing their emotions?
   - Reflection: _____

Tips:

- Compassion is key to helping firefighter parts feel supported. By showing them understanding, you create space for healthier changes.
- Focus on offering small, actionable alternatives that your firefighter parts can use in place of addictive behaviors.

Therapist Comments/Feedback:

- "Building compassion for your firefighter parts is a major step in healing. With time, they'll begin to trust that there are safer, healthier ways to manage emotional pain."

Worksheet 86: Steps for Unburdening Addictive Parts

Goal: To guide the user in unburdening the parts that engage in addictive behaviors, helping them release the emotional weight they carry.

Step 1: Identifying the Burdens Behind Addictive Behaviors

- **Instructions**: Reflect on what emotional burdens your firefighter parts are carrying that lead them to engage in addictive behaviors.

1. What burdens are your firefighter parts carrying, and how do these burdens influence their behavior?
    - Example: "My firefighter part is burdened by fear and stress, and it turns to addiction to find relief."
    - The burdens behind my firefighter parts' behaviors are: _____

Step 2: Inviting Addictive Parts to Release Their Burdens

- **Instructions**: Imagine inviting your firefighter parts to release their burdens. Let them know that they no longer have to carry the emotional weight they've been holding onto.

1. What can you say to your firefighter parts to encourage them to release their burdens?
    - Reflection: _____

Step 3: Visualizing the Unburdening Process

- **Instructions**: Close your eyes and visualize your firefighter parts releasing their burdens. Imagine these burdens being lifted away or transformed into something lighter.

1. How did your firefighter parts respond to the invitation to unburden, and how do you feel after the process?

- Reflection: _____

Tips:

- Unburdening addictive parts can take time. Be patient and supportive, allowing them to release their emotional weight when they feel ready.
- Offer regular check-ins with these parts to reinforce that they no longer need to carry their burdens alone.

Therapist Comments/Feedback:

- "Unburdening your addictive parts is a significant step in healing. Keep encouraging these parts to release their emotional weight, and you'll notice shifts in their behavior over time."

Part 13: Exercises for Self-Compassion

These worksheets in **Part 13: Exercises for Self-Compassion** help users develop compassion for their parts, themselves, and others, promoting healing, understanding, and connection. Each worksheet includes practical tips and therapist feedback to reinforce growth and self-kindness.

Developing Compassion for Parts

Worksheet 87: How to Approach Parts with Compassionate Curiosity

Goal: To guide the user in approaching their parts with compassionate curiosity, fostering deeper understanding and healing.

Step 1: Identifying a Part Needing Compassion

- **Instructions**: Think of a part in your system that feels misunderstood, hurt, or isolated. Reflect on how you usually interact with this part and whether it feels fully heard.

1. Which part of you needs more compassion and understanding right now?
    - Example: "My anxious part feels overwhelmed and often misunderstood."
    - The part that needs compassion is: _____

Step 2: Approaching the Part with Curiosity

- **Instructions**: Imagine sitting with this part, asking it questions with gentle curiosity. What does this part want you to know about its feelings, needs, and role in your system?

1. What does this part want to tell you when you approach it with curiosity?
    - Reflection: _____

Step 3: Offering Compassionate Listening

- **Instructions**: Write down how you can listen to this part without judgment or trying to change it, just acknowledging its presence and experiences.

1. How can you listen compassionately to this part?
    - Reflection: _____

Tips:

- Approach your parts with an open heart, avoiding judgment or the need to fix them immediately.
- Start with small, gentle questions to open up a compassionate dialogue.

Therapist Comments/Feedback:

- "Your willingness to approach your parts with curiosity is a powerful act of compassion. Keep practicing this to build stronger relationships with your parts."

Worksheet 88: Journaling Compassionate Conversations with Parts

Goal: To help the user journal compassionate conversations with their parts, creating a written dialogue that promotes healing and connection.

Step 1: Identifying a Part to Converse With

- **Instructions**: Choose a part that feels emotionally present right now. Reflect on its role, emotions, and how it has been interacting with your internal system.

1. Which part are you choosing to have a compassionate conversation with today?
    - Example: "I'm choosing my perfectionist part, which has been very critical lately."

- The part I'm conversing with is:
  _____

Step 2: Writing the Conversation

- **Instructions**: Start a conversation with this part in your journal. Allow the part to express its thoughts and feelings freely. Respond from your Self with compassion and understanding.

1. **Part**: "I'm trying to help you succeed, but I feel like you're not listening to me."
   Self: "I hear that you're worried about us not meeting expectations. I appreciate your efforts, and I want to work with you in a way that doesn't overwhelm us."

- Continue the dialogue, focusing on compassionate responses.

Step 3: Reflecting on the Conversation

- **Instructions**: Reflect on what you learned from this conversation and how it felt to connect with this part through compassionate writing.

1. What insights did you gain from this conversation, and how did it help the part feel heard?
   - Reflection: _____

Tips:

- Journaling can deepen the relationship with your parts, especially those that need more time to express themselves.
- Return to these conversations regularly to foster continued healing and understanding.

Therapist Comments/Feedback:

- "Your journaling practice is an excellent way to connect with your parts. Keep this dialogue open to allow them to express their needs in a safe, compassionate space."

Worksheet 89: Using Self-Compassion to Soothe Vulnerable Exiles

Goal: To help the user soothe vulnerable exiled parts by offering self-compassion, providing these parts with a sense of safety and care.

Step 1: Identifying a Vulnerable Exile

- **Instructions**: Reflect on a part that feels particularly vulnerable or hurt. This may be an exile that carries old wounds, fears, or shame.

1. Which exile feels vulnerable and in need of self-compassion?
    - Example: "My exile feels unlovable due to past rejections."
    - The vulnerable exile is: _____

Step 2: Offering Self-Compassion to the Exile

- **Instructions**: Imagine your Self offering this exile gentle compassion. Speak to it with kindness, letting it know it is seen, valued, and cared for.

1. What compassionate words can you offer this exile to soothe its pain?
    - Example: "You are worthy of love just as you are, and I'm here to support you."
    - Reflection: _____

Step 3: Reflecting on the Process

- **Instructions**: Write down how your exile responded to your self-compassion and what emotions arose during this process.

1. How did your exile feel after receiving compassion, and what did you learn from the experience?
    - Reflection: _____

Tips:

- Vulnerable exiles may need repeated assurance before they trust your Self's compassion—be patient and gentle with them.
- Creating a safe space for these parts will help them feel more comfortable opening up.

Therapist Comments/Feedback:

- "It's powerful that you're offering compassion to your most vulnerable parts. Keep reinforcing this message of love and care, and these exiles will feel more secure over time."

Worksheet 90: Practicing Self-Compassion in Daily Life

Goal: To guide the user in incorporating self-compassion into their daily life, helping them respond to challenges with kindness and understanding.

Step 1: Identifying Daily Opportunities for Self-Compassion

- **Instructions**: Think about moments in your daily life where you tend to be hard on yourself. These could be times of stress, failure, or self-doubt.
1. When do you tend to criticize or judge yourself during the day?
    - Example: "I'm hard on myself when I make mistakes at work or feel like I'm not doing enough."

- The situations where I need self-compassion are: _____

Step 2: Responding with Self-Compassion

- **Instructions**: Reflect on how you can respond to yourself with self-compassion in these moments. Write down a compassionate statement or practice you can use when you face these challenges.

1. How can you show yourself compassion in these situations?
    - Example: "I will remind myself that it's okay to make mistakes, and I'm doing the best I can."
    - Reflection: _____

Step 3: Practicing Self-Compassion Daily

- **Instructions**: Commit to practicing self-compassion each day. Write down one specific action or statement you will use to reinforce self-compassion in your daily routine.

1. What daily self-compassion practice will you commit to?
    - Reflection: _____

Tips:

- Self-compassion is a daily practice that grows over time. Start with small steps and build from there.
- Remind yourself that everyone experiences challenges—being kind to yourself during these moments is essential.

Therapist Comments/Feedback:

- "Incorporating self-compassion into your daily life will have a profound impact on your well-being. Keep practicing, and you'll notice a shift in how you relate to yourself."

Compassion for Self and Others

Worksheet 91: Balancing Compassion for Self and Parts

Goal: To help the user balance compassion for their Self and their parts, ensuring that both are nurtured and supported.

Step 1: Recognizing the Need for Balance

- **Instructions**: Reflect on how you currently balance your compassion for your parts and your Self. Are there moments when you neglect one in favor of the other?

1. How do you currently balance your compassion between your Self and your parts?
    - Example: "I often focus more on my parts and forget to care for my Self."
    - Reflection: _____

Step 2: Creating a Plan for Balanced Compassion

- **Instructions**: Write down a plan for how you can offer both your Self and your parts the compassion they need, ensuring that neither feels neglected.

1. How can you balance compassion for your Self and your parts moving forward?

- Reflection: _____

Step 3: Practicing Balanced Compassion

- **Instructions**: Choose a moment from today where you can practice balanced compassion for both your Self and your parts. Write down how you did it and what the outcome was.

1. What moment today allowed you to practice balanced compassion, and how did it feel?
    - Reflection: _____

Tips:

- Compassion for your Self and your parts should be equally important—both need your attention and care.
- Check in with your Self regularly to ensure that you're not overextending compassion to parts without nurturing your own needs.

Therapist Comments/Feedback:

- "Balancing compassion between your Self and your parts is a crucial part of healing. Keep this balance in mind as you move forward, and you'll feel more grounded in your relationships with both."

Worksheet 92: Practicing Compassion for Others Using IFS

Goal: To help the user practice compassion for others by applying IFS principles, recognizing that others have their own parts and internal struggles.

Step 1: Recognizing Others' Parts

- **Instructions**: Reflect on a recent interaction where you found it difficult to offer compassion to someone else. Try to view this person through the lens of IFS, recognizing that they, too, have parts that might be driving their behavior.

1. What parts of the other person do you think were active during your interaction?
    - Example: "I think their protector part was activated, trying to control the conversation because they felt vulnerable."
    - The parts I recognize in the other person are: _____

Step 2: Offering Compassion from Your Self

- **Instructions**: Write down how you can respond to this person from your Self with compassion, knowing that their behavior may be driven by their parts rather than their true Self.

1. How can you respond to this person with more compassion, understanding that they, too, have parts with their own needs?
    - Reflection: _____

Step 3: Practicing Compassion for Others

- **Instructions**: Choose a situation in your daily life where you can practice compassion for someone else using the IFS framework. Reflect on how it changes your interactions.

1. How did practicing compassion for the other person change your perspective or interaction?
    - Reflection: _____

Tips:

- Recognizing that others also have parts helps you practice empathy, even in challenging situations.
- Approach others with the same compassionate curiosity you offer to your own parts—this can transform your relationships.

Therapist Comments/Feedback:
- "Your effort to see others through the lens of IFS is a wonderful way to cultivate empathy. Keep practicing this, and you'll notice a deeper sense of connection and understanding with those around you."

Worksheet 93: Reflecting on Past Interactions Through a Compassionate Lens

Goal: To guide the user in reflecting on past interactions through the lens of self-compassion and compassion for others, transforming past judgments into understanding.

Step 1: Identifying a Challenging Past Interaction

- **Instructions**: Think of a past interaction where you were hard on yourself or someone else. Write down the details of the interaction and the emotions that came up.

1. What was the interaction, and how did you feel about yourself or the other person at the time?
    - Example: "I felt frustrated with myself for not standing up for myself in a disagreement with a friend."
    - The interaction I'm reflecting on is:
      _____

Step 2: Reframing the Interaction with Compassion

- **Instructions**: Reflect on how you can reframe this interaction through a compassionate lens, both for yourself and the other person. What parts were likely active, and how can you offer them compassion?

1. How can you now view this interaction with more compassion for both yourself and the other person?
   - Reflection: _____

Step 3: Letting Go of Judgment

- **Instructions**: Write down how you can let go of any self-judgment or judgment toward the other person, recognizing that both of you were acting from parts rather than your true Selves.

1. What judgments can you release, and how will this help you move forward?
   - Reflection: _____

Tips:

- Revisiting past interactions with compassion helps you release old judgments and see things from a more balanced, understanding perspective.
- This practice can be healing for both your relationship with yourself and your relationships with others.

Therapist Comments/Feedback:

- "Reflecting on past interactions through a compassionate lens is a powerful way to heal. Continue practicing this, and you'll find more peace with yourself and others."

Worksheet 94: How to Bring Self-Compassion into Challenging Situations

Goal: To help the user bring self-compassion into difficult situations, offering kindness and understanding to themselves in moments of stress, conflict, or challenge.

Step 1: Identifying a Challenging Situation

- **Instructions**: Think of a challenging situation you are currently facing or one that may arise in the near future. Reflect on how this situation makes you feel.

1. What challenging situation are you facing, and what emotions does it bring up?
    - Example: "I'm facing a conflict at work that makes me feel anxious and overwhelmed."
    - The challenging situation is: _____

Step 2: Bringing Self-Compassion into the Situation

- **Instructions**: Write down how you can bring self-compassion into this situation. What can you say to yourself to soothe your emotions and respond with kindness?

1. How can you offer yourself compassion in this situation?
    - Example: "I will remind myself that it's okay to feel anxious, and I will take breaks when I need them."
    - Reflection: _____

Step 3: Practicing Self-Compassion in Real-Time

- **Instructions**: Commit to practicing self-compassion the next time you face this challenging situation. Write down what you will do or say to yourself in the moment.

1. What is your plan for offering self-compassion during this challenging situation?
    - Reflection: _____

Tips:

- In moments of stress or conflict, take a pause to check in with yourself and offer self-compassion.
- Remember that challenges are part of life, and being kind to yourself during these times helps build resilience.

Therapist Comments/Feedback:

- "Your commitment to bringing self-compassion into difficult situations will greatly support your emotional well-being. Keep practicing, and over time, this will become a natural response."

Part 14: Mindfulness and Emotional Regulation

These worksheets in **Part 14: Mindfulness and Emotional Regulation** provide practical strategies to help users manage emotional overwhelm, regulate their parts, and practice mindfulness for emotional balance. Each worksheet includes tips and therapist feedback to support ongoing growth and emotional resilience.

Mindfulness to Access the Self

Worksheet 95: Using Mindfulness to Recognize Parts' Voices

Goal: To help the user use mindfulness practices to become aware of the different parts' voices in their internal system and differentiate them from the Self.

Step 1: Identifying Parts' Voices

- **Instructions**: Sit in a quiet space and practice mindfulness by bringing your awareness to your inner dialogue. Reflect on the voices you hear and how they differ.

1. What parts' voices do you notice when you quiet your mind, and how do they sound?
    - Example: "My critical part's voice is harsh and demanding, while my anxious part is quieter and more fearful."
    - The parts I recognize are: _____

Step 2: Differentiating Parts from the Self

- **Instructions**: Reflect on how the voice of your Self differs from the voices of your parts. Write down how you know when your Self is present.

1. How does the voice of your Self feel compared to the voices of your parts?
    - Reflection: _____

Step 3: Practicing Mindful Awareness

- **Instructions**: Practice listening to your parts with curiosity, noticing their voices without judgment or trying to change them.

1. How did mindfulness help you become more aware of your parts' voices?
    - Reflection: _____

Tips:

- Mindfulness helps you observe your inner dialogue without becoming overwhelmed by it.
- Listen for the calm, grounded presence of your Self among the voices of your parts.

Therapist Comments/Feedback:

- "Your ability to recognize your parts' voices through mindfulness is a key step in understanding your internal system. Keep practicing this awareness to strengthen your connection to your Self."

Worksheet 96: Developing a Daily Mindfulness Practice

Goal: To guide the user in establishing a daily mindfulness practice that supports emotional regulation and connection to the Self.

Step 1: Identifying When to Practice Mindfulness

- **Instructions**: Reflect on the times during your day when you feel the most stress or emotional reactivity. Write down when it would be most helpful to integrate a mindfulness practice.

1. What times of day do you feel most reactive or stressed, and when can you practice mindfulness?
    - Example: "I tend to feel stressed in the mornings, so I can practice mindfulness right after waking up."

- The best times for me to practice mindfulness are: _____

Step 2: Creating a Mindfulness Routine

- **Instructions**: Write down a simple daily mindfulness routine that you will follow. This could include breathwork, grounding, or body scans.

1. What will your daily mindfulness routine look like, and how long will it last?
    - Example: "I will practice five minutes of mindful breathing in the morning and do a body scan before bed."
    - My mindfulness routine is: _____

Step 3: Reflecting on Your Mindfulness Practice

- **Instructions**: After practicing mindfulness for a few days, reflect on how it affected your emotional state and connection to your parts.

1. How has practicing mindfulness daily impacted your emotional regulation and awareness of your parts?
    - Reflection: _____

Tips:

- Start small with your mindfulness practice—just a few minutes each day can make a big difference.
- Be consistent with your practice to build mindfulness into your daily routine.

Therapist Comments/Feedback:

- "Developing a daily mindfulness routine will help you stay grounded and connected to your Self. Keep it simple and consistent, and you'll notice its benefits over time."

Worksheet 97: Grounding Exercises to Return to the Self

Goal: To help the user practice grounding exercises that bring them back to their Self when they feel overwhelmed or disconnected.

Step 1: Recognizing When You Need Grounding

- **Instructions**: Reflect on the situations where you feel disconnected from your Self. Write down what triggers these feelings and when grounding exercises could be helpful.

1. When do you feel most disconnected from your Self, and what are your triggers?
    - Example: "I feel disconnected when I'm overwhelmed with work or when my anxious part takes over."
    - The situations that trigger disconnection are: _____

Step 2: Practicing a Grounding Exercise

- **Instructions**: Choose a grounding exercise such as focusing on your breath, feeling your feet on the ground, or using a calming object. Write down how this exercise made you feel.

1. Which grounding exercise did you choose, and how did it help you feel more connected to your Self?
    - Reflection: _____

Step 3: Reflecting on the Benefits of Grounding

- **Instructions**: Reflect on how grounding exercises help you return to your Self during moments of stress or emotional overwhelm.

1. How did grounding exercises help you reconnect with your Self during stressful situations?
    - Reflection: _____

Tips:

- Use grounding exercises as a quick way to reconnect with your Self when emotions feel overwhelming.
- Keep practicing different grounding techniques to find what works best for you.

Therapist Comments/Feedback:

- "Grounding exercises are a great tool for returning to your Self. Keep using them when you feel disconnected, and over time they'll become an automatic response to stress."

Worksheet 98: How to Use Breathwork to Soothe Reactive Parts

Goal: To help the user use breathwork to calm reactive parts and soothe intense emotional responses.

Step 1: Recognizing When Your Parts Are Reactive

- **Instructions**: Reflect on recent moments when your parts became reactive. Write down what triggered them and how breathwork could help in these situations.

1. When have your parts become reactive, and how could breathwork help calm them down?
    - Example: "My perfectionist part becomes reactive during stressful projects, and breathwork could help me relax."
    - The situations that trigger reactivity are: _____

Step 2: Practicing Breathwork

- **Instructions**: Choose a breathwork technique, such as deep belly breathing or box breathing. Practice this for a few minutes and reflect on how it affected your emotional state.

1. Which breathwork technique did you use, and how did it affect your reactive parts?
    - Reflection: _____

Step 3: Incorporating Breathwork into Daily Life

- **Instructions**: Write down a plan for how you can integrate breathwork into your daily routine, especially when your parts feel reactive.

1. How will you incorporate breathwork into your daily life to soothe reactive parts?
    - Reflection: _____

Tips:

- Breathwork is a powerful tool for calming reactive parts—practice it regularly to make it a habit.
- Experiment with different breathwork techniques to find the one that works best for you.

Therapist Comments/Feedback:

- "Breathwork is an excellent way to soothe reactive parts and stay grounded in your Self. Keep practicing, and over time, it will become a natural part of how you manage reactivity."

Mindfulness for Emotional Regulation

Worksheet 99: Identifying Triggers in Real Time

Goal: To help the user recognize emotional triggers as they happen and observe their reactions mindfully.

Step 1: Recognizing Emotional Triggers

- **Instructions**: Think about a recent situation where you were emotionally triggered. Write down what happened and how it made you feel.

1. What triggered your emotions, and how did it affect your internal system?
    - Example: "I was triggered when I received negative feedback at work, and my defensive part became reactive."
    - The emotional trigger was: _____

Step 2: Observing Your Reactions

- **Instructions**: Mindfully observe how your parts reacted to this trigger. Write down the parts that became activated and how they responded.

1. Which parts became activated by the trigger, and how did they respond?
    - Reflection: _____

Step 3: Mindfully Reflecting on Your Triggers

- **Instructions**: Reflect on how observing your reactions mindfully helped you stay connected to your Self during the triggering event.

1. How did mindfulness help you stay grounded while recognizing your emotional triggers?
    - Reflection: _____

Tips:

- Catching your emotional triggers in real time helps prevent reactivity. Mindful observation gives you space to respond from your Self.
- Practice observing your triggers without judgment—just notice them and allow them to pass.

Therapist Comments/Feedback:

- "Recognizing your emotional triggers in the moment is a powerful way to stay grounded. Keep practicing mindful observation, and it will become easier to manage your reactions."

Worksheet 100: Using Mindfulness to Reduce Emotional Reactivity

Goal: To help the user practice mindfulness to reduce emotional reactivity, creating space between triggers and responses.

Step 1: Recognizing Emotional Reactivity

- **Instructions**: Reflect on a recent situation where you felt emotionally reactive. Write down what triggered your reaction and how your parts responded.

1. What was the trigger, and how did your parts react emotionally?
    - Example: "I felt reactive when my friend criticized my decision, and my defensive part took over."
    - The emotional reactivity I experienced was: _____

Step 2: Practicing Mindfulness During Reactivity

- **Instructions**: When you notice emotional reactivity arising, take a mindful pause. Focus on your breath or body sensations to create a moment of calm before reacting.

1. How did practicing mindfulness during a reactive moment help you calm down and avoid escalation?
    - Reflection: _____

Step 3: Reflecting on Mindfulness and Emotional Control

- **Instructions**: Reflect on how mindfulness helped you reduce your emotional reactivity and gain better control over your response.

1. How has mindfulness helped you reduce reactivity and respond more calmly?
    - Reflection: _____

Tips:

- When you feel reactive, take a few mindful breaths before responding. This creates a gap between the trigger and your reaction.
- Consistent mindfulness practice helps make non-reactive responses more natural over time.

Therapist Comments/Feedback:

- "Your mindfulness practice is helping you manage reactivity. Keep pausing when emotions rise, and over time, you'll feel more in control of your responses."

Worksheet 101: Mindful Self-Reflection on Difficult Emotions

Goal: To guide the user through mindful reflection on difficult emotions, allowing space for these emotions to be experienced without judgment.

Step 1: Identifying Difficult Emotions

- **Instructions**: Think of a difficult emotion you've experienced recently. Write down the emotion and the situation that brought it up.

1. What difficult emotion did you experience, and what triggered it?
    - Example: "I felt shame when I made a mistake at work."
    - The emotion I'm reflecting on is: _____

Step 2: Observing the Emotion Mindfully

- **Instructions**: Practice sitting with this emotion mindfully. Notice where you feel it in your body and how it shifts as you focus on it.

1. Where do you feel this emotion in your body, and how does it change as you observe it?
    - Reflection: _____

Step 3: Reflecting on Your Emotional Response

- **Instructions**: Write down how observing your emotion mindfully helped you understand it better or experience it differently.

1. How did mindfulness help you approach this difficult emotion with curiosity instead of judgment?
    - Reflection: _____

Tips:

- When difficult emotions arise, pause and observe them without trying to change or judge them. Just notice how they feel in your body.
- Allow emotions to flow naturally—mindful observation can help reduce the intensity of emotional experiences.

Therapist Comments/Feedback:

- "Your ability to sit with difficult emotions mindfully is a big step toward emotional regulation. Keep practicing this approach, and it will help you process emotions more smoothly."

Worksheet 102: Practicing Emotional Regulation Using Self-Led Techniques

Goal: To help the user practice emotional regulation by applying Self-led techniques to soothe activated parts and manage difficult emotions.

Step 1: Recognizing When Emotional Regulation Is Needed

- **Instructions**: Reflect on a recent moment when your emotions felt overwhelming. Write down the emotion and how it affected your internal system.

1. What was the overwhelming emotion, and how did it affect your parts?

- Example: "I felt overwhelmed with anger during an argument, and my firefighter part wanted to escape."
- The emotion I needed to regulate was: _____

Step 2: Applying a Self-Led Technique

- **Instructions**: Choose a Self-led technique, such as breathwork, grounding, or compassionate dialogue with your parts, to help regulate your emotions.

1. Which Self-led technique did you use, and how did it help you manage your emotional state?
   - Reflection: _____

Step 3: Reflecting on Emotional Regulation

- **Instructions**: Reflect on how using a Self-led technique helped you regulate your emotions and return to a state of calm.

1. How did this Self-led technique help you regain emotional balance?
   - Reflection: _____

Tips:

- When emotions feel overwhelming, remind yourself to return to your Self and apply a technique that helps you stay calm and centered.
- Practice different emotional regulation techniques to find what works best for you.

Therapist Comments/Feedback:

- "Using Self-led techniques is a great way to stay in control during emotional highs and lows. Keep practicing these techniques, and they'll become an automatic response during difficult moments."

Managing Overwhelm

Worksheet 103: Recognizing the Role of Parts in Overwhelm

Goal: To help the user recognize which parts contribute to feelings of overwhelm and how their internal system responds to stress.

Step 1: Identifying Parts Involved in Overwhelm

- **Instructions**: Reflect on a recent moment when you felt overwhelmed. Write down which parts were activated and how they contributed to the feeling.

1. Which parts were activated during your feeling of overwhelm, and how did they respond?
   - Example: "My manager part took over, trying to organize everything, and my exile part felt scared of failing."
   - The parts involved in my overwhelm are: _____

Step 2: Observing Patterns in Overwhelm

- **Instructions**: Reflect on any patterns you notice about when and how these parts react to overwhelm. Write down your observations.

1. What patterns do you notice in how your parts react when you feel overwhelmed?

- Reflection: _____

Step 3: Reflecting on Overwhelm and Parts' Roles

- **Instructions**: Write down how recognizing your parts' roles in overwhelm has helped you understand your reactions better.

1. How has recognizing your parts' roles in overwhelm helped you better manage your stress?
    - Reflection: _____

Tips:

- Overwhelm often happens when multiple parts get activated at once. Observing which parts are involved can help you better manage their responses.
- When feeling overwhelmed, pause to check in with your parts and see what they need.

Therapist Comments/Feedback:

- "Recognizing how your parts contribute to overwhelm is a great step toward managing stress. Keep checking in with these parts, and you'll gain more control over how you handle overwhelm."

Worksheet 104: Self-Soothing Strategies for Overwhelming Situations

Goal: To guide the user in developing self-soothing strategies to calm their system during moments of overwhelm.

Step 1: Identifying Overwhelming Situations

- **Instructions**: Reflect on a recent situation where you felt overwhelmed. Write down what triggered the feeling of overwhelm and how it affected you.

1. What situation caused you to feel overwhelmed, and how did it affect your parts and emotions?
    - Example: "I felt overwhelmed by the number of tasks I had at work, and my anxious part became active."
    - The overwhelming situation I experienced was: _____

Step 2: Developing Self-Soothing Strategies

- **Instructions**: Write down a few self-soothing strategies you can use when you feel overwhelmed, such as deep breathing, grounding, or positive self-talk.

1. What self-soothing strategies can you use to calm yourself during overwhelming situations?
    - Reflection: _____

Step 3: Practicing Self-Soothing

- **Instructions**: The next time you feel overwhelmed, practice one of the self-soothing strategies and reflect on how it helped calm your system.

1. Which strategy did you use, and how did it help soothe your overwhelmed parts?
    - Reflection: _____

Tips:

- Self-soothing strategies are important for calming the nervous system during moments of overwhelm. Practice them regularly to make them part of your routine.
- Create a list of self-soothing strategies you can easily access when stress arises.

Therapist Comments/Feedback:

- "Your self-soothing strategies are a valuable tool for managing overwhelm. Keep practicing them, and they'll help you feel more grounded during stressful moments."

Worksheet 105: Emotional Regulation for Firefighter Parts

Goal: To help the user manage the emotional responses of firefighter parts, which often react to overwhelm with avoidance or impulsivity.

Step 1: Recognizing Firefighter Responses

- **Instructions**: Reflect on how your firefighter parts react when you feel overwhelmed or emotionally triggered. Write down the behaviors they use to manage the situation.

1. How do your firefighter parts react during overwhelming situations, and what behaviors do they use?
    - Example: "My firefighter part distracts me with social media when I feel overwhelmed."
    - The firefighter part's responses are:
      _____

Step 2: Offering Emotional Regulation to Firefighters

- **Instructions**: Write down a strategy you can use to help your firefighter parts regulate their emotional responses more effectively, such as grounding or self-compassion.

1. What strategy can you offer your firefighter parts to help them manage emotions without reacting impulsively?
    - Reflection: _____

Step 3: Reflecting on the Process

- **Instructions**: Reflect on how regulating your firefighter parts' responses helps reduce overwhelm and promote emotional balance.

1. How did emotional regulation strategies help calm your firefighter parts and reduce reactivity?
    - Reflection: _____

Tips:

- Firefighter parts often react quickly to stress. Offering them emotional regulation tools helps them feel more in control.
- Engage with your firefighter parts compassionately, understanding that they're trying to protect you from overwhelm.

Therapist Comments/Feedback:

- "Helping your firefighter parts regulate their emotions is a key step in managing overwhelm. Keep offering them tools to calm down, and you'll notice a shift in their responses."

Worksheet 106: Journaling Through Overwhelm

Goal: To help the user process feelings of overwhelm through journaling, providing clarity and emotional relief.

Step 1: Journaling About Overwhelm

- **Instructions**: Reflect on a recent experience of overwhelm and journal about what triggered it, how your parts reacted, and how it affected your emotional state.

1. What caused your overwhelm, and how did your parts respond to the situation?
    - Example: "I felt overwhelmed by family expectations, and my anxious part reacted by overthinking."
    - The experience of overwhelm I'm journaling about is: _____

Step 2: Exploring Solutions Through Journaling

- **Instructions**: Journal about possible solutions to manage overwhelm in the future, such as self-soothing strategies or setting boundaries.

1. What solutions can you explore to manage overwhelm more effectively next time?
    - Reflection: _____

Step 3: Reflecting on the Impact of Journaling

- **Instructions**: Write down how journaling helped you process your feelings of overwhelm and gain a clearer perspective on your emotional experience.

1. How did journaling help you feel more in control and aware of your emotional state?

- Reflection: _____

Tips:

- Journaling is a great way to process overwhelming emotions. It helps externalize your thoughts and bring clarity to the situation.
- Make journaling a regular part of your emotional regulation practice to manage stress more effectively.

Therapist Comments/Feedback:

- "Journaling is a powerful tool for processing overwhelm. Keep writing about your experiences, and you'll gain more insight into your emotions and how to handle them."

Part 15: Specialized Worksheets for Therapists

These **Part 15: Specialized Worksheets for Therapists** offer structured approaches for guiding clients through IFS work in sessions, supporting them through specific challenges like anxiety, depression, trauma, and unburdening. Each worksheet includes therapist guidance, tips, and reflection points for clients, reinforcing the therapeutic process.

For Use with Clients in Session

Worksheet 107: Helping Clients Identify Their Parts

Goal: To assist therapists in guiding clients through the process of identifying their parts, fostering self-awareness and understanding.

Step 1: Explaining the Concept of Parts

- **Instructions for Therapist**: Explain the concept of parts in a client-friendly way, helping the client understand that their different emotions and behaviors may come from distinct parts of their internal system.

1. **Therapist's Explanation**: Describe the concept of parts and how they function in the client's internal system.
    - Example: "We all have parts that take on different roles in our lives—some protect us, some help us get things done, and others carry pain."

Step 2: Helping the Client Identify Parts

- **Instructions for Therapist**: Ask the client to reflect on a recent emotional experience. Guide them to identify the parts involved in that experience and what role each part played.

1. **Client's Reflection**: What parts were involved in your recent emotional experience, and what role did each part play?
    - Reflection: _____

Step 3: Offering Feedback

- **Instructions for Therapist**: Provide feedback on the client's identification of their parts, helping them gain more clarity and insight into the dynamics of their internal system.

Tips for Therapists:

- Use simple language and metaphors when introducing the concept of parts, especially for clients who are new to IFS.

- Encourage clients to identify parts without judgment, viewing each part as trying to help in its own way.

Therapist Comments/Feedback:

- "Great work identifying your parts! Keep observing how different parts show up in various situations, and we'll continue exploring them together."

Worksheet 108: Mapping a Client's Internal System

Goal: To help therapists guide clients through mapping their internal system, visualizing how their parts interact with each other and the Self.

Step 1: Identifying Key Parts

- **Instructions for Therapist**: Ask the client to identify the key parts they interact with most frequently. Help them reflect on which parts are dominant in their internal system.

1. **Client's Reflection**: What are the main parts that come up for you in everyday life?
    - Reflection: _____

Step 2: Mapping the Relationships Between Parts

- **Instructions for Therapist**: Work with the client to create a visual map of their internal system, showing how their parts interact with each other and the Self. Focus on protector-exile dynamics, conflicts, or alliances between parts.

1. **Client's Map**: What is the relationship between your parts, and how do they interact?
     - Reflection: _____

Step 3: Offering Feedback and Support

- **Instructions for Therapist**: Provide feedback on the client's map, highlighting patterns and areas where parts may need more attention or balance.

Tips for Therapists:

- Use visual aids such as diagrams or drawings to help clients understand the relationships between their parts.
- Encourage clients to explore both protector and exile parts, helping them see the full picture of their internal system.

Therapist Comments/Feedback:

- "Your internal map shows a lot of helpful insight into how your parts are working together. We can use this map to guide our work in bringing more balance to your system."

Worksheet 109: Introducing Clients to the Concept of Self-Leadership

Goal: To help therapists introduce clients to the concept of Self-leadership, empowering them to lead their internal system with calm, curiosity, and compassion.

Step 1: Explaining Self-Leadership

- **Instructions for Therapist**: Introduce the concept of Self-leadership, explaining that the Self is the calm, compassionate core that can guide parts toward healing.

1. **Therapist's Explanation**: What does Self-leadership mean, and how does it help you guide your parts?
    - Example: "The Self is the part of you that is calm, confident, and capable of leading your internal system with compassion."

Step 2: Helping the Client Access the Self

- **Instructions for Therapist**: Guide the client through a mindfulness or visualization exercise to help them access their Self. Encourage them to feel the qualities of calm, curiosity, and compassion.

1. **Client's Reflection**: How did it feel to access your Self, and what qualities did you notice?
    - Reflection: _____

Step 3: Encouraging Self-Led Engagement with Parts

- **Instructions for Therapist**: Encourage the client to use their Self to engage with their parts, offering compassion and leadership to any parts in distress.

Tips for Therapists:

- Use simple exercises like grounding or breathwork to help clients access their Self.
- Remind clients that Self-leadership isn't about perfection—it's about leading with compassion and curiosity.

Therapist Comments/Feedback:

- "You're doing an amazing job accessing your Self. Keep practicing this, and you'll notice how your Self can guide your parts with more ease."

Worksheet 110: Exploring Client's Firefighters and Protectors

Goal: To help therapists guide clients in exploring their firefighter and protector parts, understanding how these parts try to manage pain and emotional distress.

Step 1: Identifying Firefighter and Protector Parts

- **Instructions for Therapist**: Ask the client to reflect on how they cope with emotional pain or stress. Guide them to identify the firefighter and protector parts that take on this role.

1. **Client's Reflection**: What firefighter or protector parts come up when you feel emotionally overwhelmed or distressed?
    - Example: "My firefighter part distracts me with work when I feel anxious."
    - Reflection: _____

Step 2: Exploring the Role of Firefighters and Protectors

- **Instructions for Therapist**: Help the client understand what these parts are trying to achieve. Are they protecting exiled parts, managing emotions, or avoiding pain?

1. **Client's Reflection**: What are your firefighters and protectors trying to achieve?
    - Reflection: _____

Step 3: Offering Compassion to Firefighters and Protectors

- **Instructions for Therapist**: Encourage the client to approach their firefighter and protector parts with compassion, recognizing that these parts are trying to help, even if their methods aren't always healthy.

Tips for Therapists:

- Help clients understand that firefighter and protector parts are working to manage pain, even if they engage in unhealthy behaviors.
- Encourage clients to offer compassion and curiosity to these parts, helping them feel seen and understood.

Therapist Comments/Feedback:

- "It's great that you're recognizing your firefighter and protector parts. By offering them compassion, you can start to change their behavior and help them feel more supported."

For Supporting Clients with Specific Issues

Worksheet 111: Working with Clients Who Have Anxiety

Goal: To help therapists guide clients through identifying anxiety-related parts and offering Self-led strategies to manage anxiety.

Step 1: Identifying Anxiety-Related Parts

- **Instructions for Therapist**: Ask the client to reflect on moments when they feel anxious. Help them identify which parts become active during anxiety, and what role each part plays.

1. **Client's Reflection**: What parts are activated when you feel anxious, and how do they react?
   - Reflection: _____

Step 2: Developing Self-Led Anxiety Management Strategies

- **Instructions for Therapist**: Guide the client in developing Self-led techniques, such as mindfulness or grounding, to help soothe anxious parts.

1. **Client's Reflection**: What Self-led strategies can help you manage your anxiety?
   - Reflection: _____

Step 3: Offering Feedback and Encouragement

- **Instructions for Therapist**: Offer feedback on the client's progress, helping them refine their anxiety management strategies.

Tips for Therapists:

- Encourage clients to practice self-compassion when managing anxiety. Remind them that anxious parts are often trying to protect them.
- Use mindfulness and grounding techniques to help clients reconnect with their Self during anxious moments.

Therapist Comments/Feedback:

- "You're doing great identifying your anxiety-related parts. Keep practicing your Self-led strategies, and over time, your anxious parts will feel more supported."

Worksheet 112: Guiding Clients Through Depression Work

Goal: To help therapists guide clients through identifying and working with parts related to depression, offering Self-led techniques to support healing.

Step 1: Identifying Depression-Related Parts

- **Instructions for Therapist**: Ask the client to reflect on moments when they feel depressed or hopeless. Help them identify which parts carry these feelings of depression.

1. **Client's Reflection**: What parts come up when you feel depressed, and how do they express these feelings?
    - Example: "My exiled part holds sadness from past experiences of rejection."
    - Reflection: _____

Step 2: Exploring the Root of Depression

- **Instructions for Therapist**: Help the client explore the origin of these depression-related parts, focusing on when and why these parts first started carrying their burdens.

1. **Client's Reflection**: When did these parts start carrying depression, and what triggered these emotions?
    - Reflection: _____

Step 3: Offering Compassion to Depression-Related Parts

- **Instructions for Therapist**: Guide the client in offering compassion and support to their depression-related parts, helping them feel seen and understood.

Tips for Therapists:

- Encourage clients to approach their depression-related parts with gentleness, recognizing that these parts are often burdened by long-held emotional pain.
- Use visualizations or grounding exercises to help clients soothe their depression-related parts.

Therapist Comments/Feedback:

- "You're making important strides in recognizing your depression-related parts. By offering them compassion, you're creating a safe space for healing."

Worksheet 113: Trauma-Informed Unburdening for Clients

Goal: To help therapists guide clients through the trauma-informed unburdening process, ensuring emotional safety and healing.

Step 1: Identifying Trauma-Related Burdens

- **Instructions for Therapist**: Ask the client to reflect on a specific trauma and identify the parts that carry the emotional burden of this trauma.

1. **Client's Reflection**: Which parts are holding the burden of trauma, and what emotions are they carrying?
    - Example: "My exiled part holds fear and shame from a childhood experience."
    - Reflection: _____

Step 2: Preparing for Unburdening

- **Instructions for Therapist**: Guide the client through creating emotional safety before unburdening trauma-related parts. This might involve mindfulness, grounding, or creating a safe internal space.

1. **Client's Reflection**: How can you create safety before unburdening your trauma-related parts?
    - Reflection: _____

Step 3: Guiding the Unburdening Process

- **Instructions for Therapist**: Gently guide the client in visualizing their trauma-related parts releasing their burdens. Encourage them to offer their parts compassion during this process.

Tips for Therapists:

- Always prioritize emotional safety when working with trauma-related parts. Use grounding techniques to ensure the client feels supported.
- Move at the client's pace, allowing them to unburden trauma when they feel ready.

Therapist Comments/Feedback:

- "You're doing an incredible job preparing your parts for unburdening. Keep focusing on emotional safety, and the unburdening process will unfold naturally."

Worksheet 114: Building Emotional Safety Before Addressing Trauma

Goal: To help therapists guide clients in building emotional safety before addressing trauma, ensuring they feel grounded and secure during trauma work.

Step 1: Recognizing the Need for Emotional Safety

- **Instructions for Therapist**: Help the client reflect on why emotional safety is important before addressing trauma. Guide them to identify situations where they may feel unsafe.

1. **Client's Reflection**: Why is emotional safety important when addressing trauma, and in what situations do you feel unsafe?
    - Reflection: _____

Step 2: Creating Emotional Safety

- **Instructions for Therapist**: Guide the client in creating emotional safety through grounding exercises, breathwork, or visualizing a safe internal space.

1. **Client's Reflection**: What grounding or safety techniques help you feel safe before addressing trauma?
    - Reflection: _____

Step 3: Maintaining Safety During Trauma Work

- **Instructions for Therapist**: Encourage the client to use safety techniques throughout their trauma work, ensuring that they feel supported and secure.

Tips for Therapists:

- Before addressing trauma, help the client establish emotional safety with grounding techniques, calming visualizations, or breathwork.
- Encourage clients to take breaks during trauma work if they feel overwhelmed, and always prioritize their sense of safety.

Therapist Comments/Feedback:

- "You're doing excellent work creating emotional safety. Keep using these techniques whenever you approach trauma, and it will help you feel more secure throughout the process."

Guided IFS Sessions

Worksheet 115: Step-by-Step Guide to Conducting a Parts Exploration Session

Goal: To help therapists guide clients through an IFS parts exploration session, identifying and engaging with different parts.

Step 1: Setting the Intention for the Session

- **Instructions for Therapist**: Begin by asking the client to set an intention for the session. What part do they want to explore today?

1. **Client's Intention**: What part would you like to explore during today's session, and what is your goal?
    - Reflection: _____

Step 2: Exploring the Part

- **Instructions for Therapist**: Guide the client through engaging with the part they wish to explore. Encourage them to ask the part what it needs and what role it plays.

1. **Client's Reflection**: What does this part want to tell you, and what role does it play in your system?
    - Reflection: _____

Step 3: Offering Support to the Part

- **Instructions for Therapist**: Help the client offer support and understanding to the part, listening to its needs and offering compassion from the Self.

Tips for Therapists:

- Start the session by setting a clear intention with the client, ensuring they feel focused and prepared for the exploration.
- Encourage the client to approach their part with curiosity, helping them build a compassionate dialogue with the part.

Therapist Comments/Feedback:

- "Your parts exploration is going really well. Keep engaging with your parts with curiosity and compassion, and you'll continue to build stronger internal relationships."

Worksheet 116: Helping Clients Offer Compassion to Their Parts

Goal: To help therapists guide clients in offering compassion to their parts, fostering healing and self-compassion.

Step 1: Identifying a Part That Needs Compassion

- **Instructions for Therapist**: Ask the client to reflect on a part that feels distressed, misunderstood, or burdened. Guide them to identify this part and recognize its needs.

1. **Client's Reflection**: Which part feels in need of compassion, and what burden is it carrying?
    - Reflection: _____

Step 2: Offering Compassion to the Part

- **Instructions for Therapist**: Guide the client in offering compassion to the part, speaking to it with kindness and understanding. Encourage the client to acknowledge the part's pain.

1. **Client's Reflection**: What compassionate message can you offer to this part?
    - Reflection: _____

Step 3: Reflecting on the Process

- **Instructions for Therapist**: Help the client reflect on how offering compassion to their part affected the part and their internal system as a whole.

Tips for Therapists:

- Encourage clients to offer compassion to parts that may feel hurt or burdened. Compassion helps parts feel seen and understood.
- Use visualization techniques to help clients connect with their parts on a deeper emotional level.

Therapist Comments/Feedback:

- "You're doing wonderful work offering compassion to your parts. Keep practicing this, and it will deepen your connection with them and promote healing."

Worksheet 117: Creating Safe Visualizations for Exiles

Goal: To help therapists guide clients in creating safe visualizations for exiled parts, offering these parts a space to feel protected and understood.

Step 1: Identifying an Exile in Need of Safety

- **Instructions for Therapist**: Ask the client to reflect on an exiled part that feels vulnerable or unsafe. Help them identify this part and acknowledge its need for safety.

1. **Client's Reflection**: Which exiled part feels vulnerable, and how does it need safety?
    - Reflection: _____

Step 2: Creating a Safe Visualization for the Exile

- **Instructions for Therapist**: Guide the client in creating a safe internal space for their exiled part. This might be a peaceful, protected environment where the exile can feel secure.

1. **Client's Reflection**: What does the safe space you've created for your exile look like, and how does it make your exile feel?
    - Reflection: _____

Step 3: Reflecting on the Safety Process

- **Instructions for Therapist**: Encourage the client to reflect on how creating this safe space affected their exile and the overall system.

Tips for Therapists:

- When creating safe visualizations, encourage the client to engage their senses—help them imagine what the space looks, feels, and sounds like.
- Use grounding exercises before the visualization to help the client feel calm and centered.

Therapist Comments/Feedback:

- "The safe space you've created for your exiled part is beautiful. Keep using this visualization to help your exile feel secure and protected."

Worksheet 118: Techniques for Unburdening During a Session

Goal: To help therapists guide clients through the unburdening process during a session, facilitating the release of emotional burdens.

Step 1: Preparing for Unburdening

- **Instructions for Therapist**: Ask the client to identify a part that is ready to unburden. Guide them in preparing the part emotionally, ensuring it feels safe and supported.

1. **Client's Reflection**: Which part is ready to unburden, and how can you ensure its safety during the process?
    - Reflection: _____

Step 2: Facilitating the Unburdening Process

- **Instructions for Therapist**: Guide the client through visualizing the part releasing its burden. Encourage the client to offer compassion and understanding as the part lets go of its weight.

1. **Client's Reflection**: How did the unburdening process feel, and how did the part respond to it?
    - Reflection: _____

Step 3: Reflecting on the Unburdening

- **Instructions for Therapist**: Encourage the client to reflect on how the unburdening process affected their internal system and what changes they noticed after the session.

Tips for Therapists:

- Take time to prepare the client's part for unburdening, ensuring that it feels safe and ready to let go of its emotional burden.
- Move slowly through the unburdening process, allowing the client to feel fully supported throughout.

Therapist Comments/Feedback:

- "You did an excellent job guiding your part through the unburdening process. Keep offering it compassion and support, and it will continue to heal."

Part 16: Worksheets for Stages of IFS Work

These worksheets in **Part 16: Stages of IFS Work** are designed to guide users through various stages of IFS practice, from beginner to advanced. Each worksheet provides practical steps, tips, and therapist feedback to support the user's journey through identifying, healing, and reintegrating parts, with a strong emphasis on self-compassion and trauma healing at the advanced level.

Beginner Worksheets

Worksheet 119: Identifying Your First Protector Part

Goal: To help beginners identify their first protector part, fostering awareness of how this part plays a role in managing their internal system.

Step 1: Reflecting on Protectors

- **Instructions**: Think about situations where you feel the need to control or protect yourself emotionally. These moments often signal the presence of a protector part. Write down an example from your recent experiences.

1. What situation made you feel the need to protect yourself, and how did you react?
    - Example: "When I felt criticized at work, I became defensive and tried to explain myself quickly."
    - Reflection: _____

Step 2: Recognizing Your Protector Part

- **Instructions**: Reflect on which part of you was active in this situation. What role did this part play, and how was it trying to help?

1. Which part was trying to protect you, and what was its goal?
    - Reflection: _____

Step 3: Offering Curiosity to Your Protector

- **Instructions**: Approach this protector part with curiosity. Write down what you think this part would say if you asked it why it acted the way it did.

1. What do you think your protector part would say if it could explain its actions?
    - Reflection: _____

Tips:

- Your protector parts often take action to shield you from pain or vulnerability. Approach them with curiosity rather than judgment.
- Starting to recognize these parts is the first step toward building a compassionate relationship with them.

Therapist Comments/Feedback:

- "Great job identifying your protector part. Keep noticing when it comes up, and remember to approach it with understanding and curiosity."

Worksheet 120: Understanding Firefighters' Roles in Stress Management

Goal: To help beginners understand how firefighter parts manage stress by distracting, soothing, or avoiding emotional pain.

Step 1: Identifying Firefighter Responses

- **Instructions**: Think of a time when you felt overwhelmed or stressed. Reflect on how you reacted to manage this stress, and identify any behaviors that helped you escape or avoid the feelings.

1. What stressful situation did you face, and how did you manage the feelings that came up?
    - Example: "I felt overwhelmed by a deadline, so I distracted myself by binge-watching TV shows."
    - Reflection: _____

Step 2: Recognizing Firefighter Behaviors

- **Instructions**: Write down which part of you engaged in distraction or avoidance during this stressful moment. Reflect on how it was trying to protect you.

1. What firefighter part was activated during this stressful moment, and how did it try to help you avoid pain?
    - Reflection: _____

Step 3: Offering Compassion to Firefighters

- **Instructions**: Approach your firefighter part with understanding. Write down how you might offer it compassion, recognizing that it is trying to help.

1. How can you offer compassion to this firefighter part, knowing that it's doing its best to protect you?
    - Reflection: _____

Tips:

- Firefighter parts often use distraction or avoidance to protect you from intense emotions. Acknowledge their role with compassion.
- Learning to recognize these parts is key to understanding your stress management patterns.

Therapist Comments/Feedback:

- "Your insight into how your firefighter part handles stress is a great step. Keep offering it compassion as you learn more about how it operates."

Worksheet 121: Simple Grounding Exercises for Beginners

Goal: To help beginners practice basic grounding exercises that bring them back to the Self when feeling overwhelmed.

Step 1: Recognizing the Need for Grounding

- **Instructions**: Think about moments when you felt emotionally overwhelmed or disconnected from yourself. Write down a recent experience where you felt this way.

1. What situation made you feel overwhelmed or disconnected from yourself?
    - Reflection: _____

Step 2: Practicing a Simple Grounding Exercise

- **Instructions**: Try one of these simple grounding techniques:
    - Take five deep breaths, focusing on the sensation of air entering and leaving your body.
    - Feel your feet on the ground and notice how they make contact with the earth.
    - Name five things you can see around you to bring your attention back to the present.

1. Which grounding technique did you try, and how did it help you feel more connected to the present moment?

- Reflection: _____

Step 3: Reflecting on the Experience

- **Instructions**: Write down how practicing grounding affected your emotional state and sense of connection to your Self.

1. How did grounding help you feel more calm and centered?
   - Reflection: _____

Tips:

- Grounding exercises are simple yet powerful tools to help you return to the present moment and reconnect with your Self.
- Practice grounding regularly, even when you're not overwhelmed, to build this skill over time.

Therapist Comments/Feedback:

- "You did great practicing grounding. Keep using these techniques when you feel disconnected, and they'll become a natural part of how you manage stress."

Worksheet 122: Beginner's Guide to Mapping Your Internal System

Goal: To help beginners create a simple map of their internal system, identifying key parts and understanding how they interact.

Step 1: Identifying Key Parts

- **Instructions**: Start by identifying a few key parts that show up regularly in your life. Write down their roles and how they affect your emotions or behaviors.

1. What are the main parts that show up in your daily life, and what are their roles?

    o   Reflection: _____

Step 2: Creating Your Internal System Map

- **Instructions**: Draw a simple map of your internal system, showing how your parts relate to each other. You can use circles to represent parts and lines to show relationships between them (e.g., conflicts, cooperation).

1. What did you notice about the relationships between your parts as you created this map?

    o   Reflection: _____

Step 3: Reflecting on Your Internal System

- **Instructions**: Write down what you learned from mapping your internal system and how it helped you understand your parts better.

1. How has mapping your system helped you see your parts and their roles more clearly?

    o   Reflection: _____

Tips:

- Mapping your internal system is a powerful way to visualize how your parts work together. You don't have to be an artist—simple shapes and lines work great.

- As you explore more parts, you can continue to expand your map.

Therapist Comments/Feedback:

- "Your internal system map is a great start! Keep adding to it as you discover more parts and notice how their relationships evolve."

Intermediate Worksheets

Worksheet 123: Exploring Conflict Between Parts

Goal: To help intermediate-level users identify and explore conflicts between parts, fostering a deeper understanding of internal struggles.

Step 1: Identifying Conflicting Parts

- **Instructions**: Reflect on a recent internal conflict you experienced. This might involve a part of you wanting to do something while another part resisted. Write down the situation and the parts involved.

1. What was the situation, and which parts were in conflict?
    - Example: "I wanted to rest, but my perfectionist part felt guilty about not working."
    - The conflicting parts are: _____

Step 2: Understanding the Needs of Each Part

- **Instructions**: Take a moment to listen to each part. What does each part want or need? Why are they acting the way they are? Write down their perspectives.

1. What does each part want, and why is it in conflict with the other part?
    - Reflection: _____

Step 3: Offering Compassion to Both Parts

- **Instructions**: Approach each part with compassion, recognizing that both are trying to help you in their own way. Write down how you can offer understanding and support to each part.

1. How can you offer compassion and support to each conflicting part?

- Reflection: _____

Tips:

- Internal conflicts often arise from parts trying to protect or help you in different ways. Listening to both sides helps you resolve these conflicts.
- Approach both parts with curiosity and empathy, knowing that neither part is "bad"—they just have different goals.

Therapist Comments/Feedback:

- "You're doing a great job exploring the conflict between your parts. Keep listening to their needs, and over time, you'll find ways to help them work together."

Worksheet 124: Understanding How Exiles Affect Daily Life

Goal: To help intermediate-level users recognize how their exiled parts affect their daily life and emotional experiences.

Step 1: Identifying an Exiled Part

- **Instructions**: Reflect on a part of you that carries pain, fear, or shame—this is likely an exiled part. Write down how this part affects your emotions or behaviors in daily life.

1. Which exiled part affects your daily life, and how does it manifest?
   - Example: "My exiled part carries shame from a past rejection, and it makes me feel unworthy in relationships."
   - The exiled part is: _____

Step 2: Recognizing the Impact of the Exile

- **Instructions**: Write down specific examples of how this exiled part's pain influences your interactions, emotions, or decisions.

1. How does this exile's pain affect your daily life and emotional experiences?
    - Reflection: _____

Step 3: Offering Compassion to the Exile

- **Instructions**: Approach your exiled part with compassion. Write down how you can offer this part a sense of safety, understanding, and support.

1. How can you offer compassion and safety to this exiled part?
    - Reflection: _____

Tips:

- Exiled parts often carry deep emotional burdens that can affect how you feel and behave. Acknowledging their impact is the first step in healing.
- Approach your exiled parts with care, understanding that their pain is likely rooted in past experiences.

Therapist Comments/Feedback:

- "You're doing important work by recognizing how your exiled parts influence your daily life. Keep offering them compassion and safety, and you'll start to see shifts in how they affect you."

Worksheet 125: Balancing Multiple Protectors in Your System

Goal: To help intermediate-level users explore how multiple protector parts interact and learn to balance their roles within the system.

Step 1: Identifying Multiple Protectors

- **Instructions**: Reflect on a situation where you felt different protector parts were active at the same time. Write down how each protector part responded and what its role was.

1. What situation triggered multiple protectors, and how did each one respond?
    - Example: "I felt pressure at work, so my organizer part took over, while my perfectionist part added more stress."
    - The protector parts involved are:
      _____

Step 2: Understanding the Roles of Each Protector

- **Instructions**: Write down the role of each protector part and what it is trying to achieve in the system. Notice if any protectors are in conflict with each other.

1. What role does each protector part play, and are they in conflict?
    - Reflection: _____

Step 3: Finding Balance Between Protectors

- **Instructions**: Reflect on how you can help your protector parts work together harmoniously, ensuring that no part feels overburdened.

1. How can you help your protector parts balance their roles and work together?
    - Reflection: _____

Tips:

- Protector parts may have different goals or strategies, which can create internal tension. Help them find balance by recognizing and respecting their roles.
- Use Self-leadership to guide protector parts, ensuring they don't take on too much responsibility.

Therapist Comments/Feedback:

- "Balancing multiple protectors is a key part of IFS work. You're doing great by helping them work together without overwhelming the system."

Worksheet 126: Unburdening Exiles for Intermediate IFS Practitioners

Goal: To guide intermediate-level users through the process of unburdening exiled parts in a safe and compassionate way.

Step 1: Identifying an Exile Ready for Unburdening

- **Instructions**: Reflect on an exiled part that feels ready to release its burdens. Write down what emotional burdens this part has been carrying and why it is ready to let go.

1. Which exiled part is ready for unburdening, and what emotional burdens is it carrying?
    - Example: "My exiled part carries the fear of abandonment, and it feels ready to release this burden."
    - The exiled part is: _____

Step 2: Preparing for Unburdening

- **Instructions**: Before unburdening, create a safe internal space for your exile. Visualize a peaceful place where it can feel secure during the process.

1. What safe space have you created for your exile, and how does it make the part feel?
    - Reflection: _____

Step 3: Guiding the Unburdening Process

- **Instructions**: Gently guide your exile through the unburdening process. Imagine it releasing its emotional burdens in a way that feels natural, such as letting go of heavy weights or transforming dark energy into light.

1. How did the unburdening process feel, and how did the exile respond?
    - Reflection: _____

Tips:

- Unburdening is a powerful process that requires emotional safety. Take your time, ensuring that your exile feels ready and supported.
- Visualizations can help make the unburdening process more tangible and healing for your exiled parts.

Therapist Comments/Feedback:

- "Your work on unburdening your exiled parts is deeply healing. Keep offering them compassion and safety, and their burdens will continue to lighten."

Advanced Worksheets

Worksheet 127: Advanced Visualization Techniques for Parts Healing

Goal: To help advanced IFS practitioners use complex visualization techniques to facilitate deep healing for their parts.

Step 1: Identifying a Part Needing Advanced Healing

- **Instructions**: Reflect on a part that requires deeper healing. Write down what this part is struggling with and why advanced visualization might be helpful.

1. Which part needs advanced healing, and what is it struggling with?
    - Example: "My exiled part is holding onto deep grief, and I think advanced visualization could help."
    - Reflection: _____

Step 2: Creating a Complex Visualization

- **Instructions**: Use an advanced visualization technique, such as visualizing a healing light, sending love to the part, or imagining the part in a protective environment. Write down the technique you used and how it helped.

1. What visualization technique did you use, and how did it help the part feel more healed?
    - Reflection: _____

Step 3: Reflecting on the Healing Process

- **Instructions**: Write down how the part responded to the visualization and how it affected your overall internal system.

1. How did this advanced visualization help your part heal, and what shifts did you notice in your internal system?
    - Reflection: _____

Tips:

- Advanced visualization techniques allow you to engage deeply with your parts, facilitating profound healing.
- Let your intuition guide you when creating complex visualizations—trust that your Self knows what your parts need.

Therapist Comments/Feedback:

- "You're doing incredible work using advanced visualizations. Keep trusting your Self to guide the healing process, and you'll continue to make powerful shifts."

Worksheet 128: Complex Trauma Work Using IFS

Goal: To guide advanced IFS practitioners through complex trauma work, focusing on deep healing for trauma-related parts.

Step 1: Identifying Trauma-Related Parts

- **Instructions**: Reflect on parts of your system that carry deep trauma. Write down how this trauma affects your parts and what emotions are tied to the trauma.

1. Which parts hold trauma, and how does this affect your emotional system?
    - Example: "My exile holds fear and shame from past trauma, and it causes me to feel disconnected in relationships."
    - Reflection: _____

Step 2: Creating Emotional Safety for Trauma Work

- **Instructions**: Before engaging in trauma work, ensure your parts feel emotionally safe. Visualize a protective environment or use grounding exercises to create stability.

1. What safety measures have you put in place to create emotional security for your trauma-related parts?
    - Reflection: _____

Step 3: Beginning the Trauma Healing Process

- **Instructions**: Begin engaging with your trauma-related parts, using compassion, safety, and support to help them release the emotional pain associated with trauma.

1. How did your trauma-related parts respond to the healing process, and what shifts did you notice?
    - Reflection: _____

Tips:

- Complex trauma work requires a deep sense of safety and trust. Move slowly and gently with your trauma-related parts, allowing them to release their pain over time.
- Use advanced techniques such as visualizations, unburdening, and grounding to support the healing process.

Therapist Comments/Feedback:

- "Your ability to engage in complex trauma work shows incredible courage and resilience. Keep offering your parts safety and compassion, and their healing will continue."

Worksheet 129: Advanced Self-Compassion Techniques for Trauma Survivors

Goal: To help advanced IFS practitioners use deep self-compassion techniques to support trauma recovery, building a compassionate connection with exiled and protector parts.

Step 1: Identifying Parts in Need of Deep Compassion

- **Instructions**: Reflect on parts of your system, especially those related to trauma, that need advanced levels of self-compassion. Write down which parts feel burdened by pain or fear and how this affects your system.

1. Which parts are carrying trauma-related burdens, and how does their pain impact your life?
    - Example: "My exile holds guilt from past trauma, and it makes me feel unworthy in relationships."
    - Reflection: _____

Step 2: Practicing Advanced Self-Compassion

- **Instructions**: Use a deep self-compassion technique, such as speaking to your parts with profound kindness, visualizing yourself offering unconditional love, or embracing your parts with soothing energy. Write down the technique you used and how it felt.

1. Which self-compassion technique did you use, and how did it impact your parts?
    - Reflection: _____

Step 3: Reflecting on the Healing Process

- **Instructions**: Write down how practicing advanced self-compassion affected your trauma-related parts and your internal system overall.

1. How did deep self-compassion help your parts release their burdens, and what shifts did you notice?

    o   Reflection: _____

Tips:

- Trauma-related parts often need deep levels of self-compassion to begin healing. Speak to them with love, patience, and care.
- Advanced self-compassion techniques can help shift deeply embedded feelings of shame, guilt, or unworthiness.

Therapist Comments/Feedback:

- "Your practice of deep self-compassion is vital for healing trauma. Keep offering this level of love and understanding to your parts, and you'll notice profound shifts in your healing process."

Worksheet 130: Integrating Unburdened Parts Into Your System

Goal: To help advanced IFS practitioners reintegrate unburdened parts into their internal system, ensuring harmony and balance after unburdening.

Step 1: Reflecting on Recently Unburdened Parts

- **Instructions**: Reflect on a part of your system that has recently gone through the unburdening process. Write down what burdens it released and how it feels now.

1. Which part did you unburden, and what emotional weights did it let go of?

- Example: "My exile released the burden of fear, and it feels lighter and more hopeful."
- Reflection: _____

Step 2: Reintegrating the Part Into the System

- **Instructions**: Focus on reintegrating the unburdened part into your internal system. Visualize this part being welcomed by other parts, establishing a new, healthier role. Write down how this process unfolded.

1. How are you reintegrating this part into your system, and how does it fit into its new role?
    - Reflection: _____

Step 3: Ensuring Balance in the System

- **Instructions**: Reflect on how your internal system is adjusting to the newly unburdened part. Write down any shifts you've noticed and how you are ensuring balance among all parts.

1. What changes have you noticed in your system since reintegrating the unburdened part, and how are you ensuring harmony?
    - Reflection: _____

Tips:

- Reintegration is a crucial part of the healing process. Make sure your unburdened part feels supported by other parts of the system.
- After unburdening, continue to check in with this part, ensuring it feels stable in its new, healthier role.

Therapist Comments/Feedback:

- "Reintegrating your unburdened parts is a key part of the healing process. Keep nurturing these parts as they adjust to their new roles, and your system will feel more balanced and whole."

Part 17: Emotional Regulation in Relationships

These worksheets in Part 17: Emotional Regulation in Relationships help guide parents and couples through the process of using IFS to navigate conflicts, foster emotional safety, and lead from the Self in relationships. Each worksheet includes practical exercises, tips, and therapist feedback to deepen emotional connection and promote healing in family and couple dynamics.

IFS for Couples

Worksheet 131: Understanding Parts in Relationship Conflicts

Goal: To help couples identify and understand the parts that are active during relationship conflicts, promoting awareness and empathy.

Step 1: Identifying Parts in Conflict

- **Instructions**: Reflect on a recent argument or disagreement in your relationship. Write down which parts of you were activated during the conflict and what role they played.

1. What disagreement did you have, and which parts were active on your side during the conflict?
    - Example: "My protector part got defensive when I felt criticized."
    - The parts activated in conflict are: _____

Step 2: Understanding Your Partner's Parts

- **Instructions**: Take time to think about which parts of your partner were activated during the conflict. Write down how you think their parts reacted and why.

1. What parts of your partner do you think were activated, and what role did they play?
    - Reflection: _____

Step 3: Offering Compassion to Both Sides

- **Instructions**: Approach both your parts and your partner's parts with compassion. Recognize that both sets of parts were trying to protect or help.

1. How can you offer compassion to your parts and your partner's parts after the conflict?
    - Reflection: _____

Tips:

- Recognize that conflicts often arise because parts are trying to protect vulnerabilities. Understanding your own parts helps bring clarity to these conflicts.
- Approach relationship conflicts with curiosity rather than blame—ask yourself what your parts were trying to protect.

Therapist Comments/Feedback:

- "Great work recognizing the parts involved in your conflict. Keep approaching these moments with compassion, and you'll notice more empathy and understanding between you and your partner."

Worksheet 132: Mapping Parts That Impact Your Relationship

Goal: To help couples create a map of the parts that influence their relationship, improving communication and connection.

Step 1: Identifying Key Parts in the Relationship

- **Instructions**: Think about the parts of you that often come up in your relationship. Write down each part's role and how it affects your interactions with your partner.

1. Which parts of you often show up in your relationship, and what role do they play?
    - Example: "My organizer part takes over when I feel like things are out of control."
    - The key parts in my relationship are: _____

Step 2: Mapping the Relationship Dynamics

- **Instructions**: Create a visual map showing how your parts interact with your partner's parts. Use lines to indicate connections, conflicts, or harmonies between the parts.

1. How do your parts interact with your partner's parts, and what patterns do you notice?
    - Reflection: _____

Step 3: Reflecting on the Map

- **Instructions**: Write down what you learned from mapping the parts in your relationship and how it can help you improve communication and emotional connection.

1. What insights did you gain from mapping your relationship dynamics?
    - Reflection: _____

Tips:

- Mapping your relationship dynamics helps you see patterns that might be hidden during conflicts. Use this map to understand each other better.
- Update your map as you explore new parts or notice changes in your relationship dynamics.

Therapist Comments/Feedback:

- "Your relationship map provides valuable insight into how your parts interact. Use this as a tool to foster deeper communication and mutual understanding."

Worksheet 133: Helping Each Other Soothe Protector Parts

Goal: To help couples learn how to soothe each other's protector parts, building trust and emotional safety in the relationship.

Step 1: Recognizing Protector Parts

- **Instructions**: Think about moments in your relationship when your protector parts become active. Write down how your protector part reacts and what it is trying to protect.

1. When does your protector part become active, and what is it trying to protect?
    - Example: "My protector part gets defensive when I feel like my opinion isn't valued."
    - Reflection: _____

Step 2: Learning How to Soothe Your Partner's Protector Parts

- **Instructions**: Ask your partner how you can help soothe their protector parts when they become activated. Write down the strategies you can use to help them feel more at ease.

1. How can you help soothe your partner's protector parts when they feel activated?
    - Reflection: _____

Step 3: Practicing Soothe Techniques

- **Instructions**: The next time your partner's protector part becomes active, practice the soothing strategies. Reflect on how it impacted the situation and their emotional state.

1. How did soothing your partner's protector part change the interaction?
    - Reflection: _____

Tips:

- Soothe each other's protector parts with empathy and patience, understanding that these parts are trying to protect vulnerabilities.
- Ask your partner directly what helps them feel safe and calm during moments of conflict or stress.

Therapist Comments/Feedback:

- "Your ability to help each other soothe protector parts is a powerful way to build emotional safety. Keep practicing these strategies to foster deeper trust and connection."

Worksheet 134: How to Lead From the Self in Relationship Conflict

Goal: To guide couples in leading from their Self during conflicts, promoting calm, compassionate communication.

Step 1: Identifying When to Lead From the Self

- **Instructions**: Reflect on a recent conflict where you didn't lead from your Self. Write down which parts took over and what the outcome was.

1. What conflict occurred, and which parts took over instead of your Self?

- Reflection: _____

Step 2: Practicing Self-Led Communication

- **Instructions**: The next time you feel a conflict arising, pause and connect with your Self before responding. Practice Self-led communication, focusing on calm, curiosity, and compassion.

1. How did leading from your Self change the way you handled the conflict?
   - Reflection: _____

Step 3: Reflecting on the Process

- **Instructions**: Write down how leading from the Self affected your emotional state and the outcome of the conflict.

1. How did leading from your Self impact the conflict and your relationship overall?
   - Reflection: _____

Tips:

- Leading from the Self requires mindfulness and patience. Practice pausing before responding to conflict and check in with your Self to ensure you're leading with calm and compassion.

- Encourage your partner to do the same, creating a space for mutual understanding during conflicts.

Therapist Comments/Feedback:

- "Leading from your Self during conflict is a transformative practice for your relationship. Keep focusing on calm, compassionate communication, and you'll notice a shift in how conflicts are resolved."

IFS for Parenting

Worksheet 135: Identifying Your Parenting Parts

Goal: To help parents identify the parts that are active in their parenting roles, improving self-awareness and connection with their children.

Step 1: Recognizing Your Parenting Parts

- **Instructions**: Reflect on the different parts of you that show up in your parenting. Write down which parts are active in specific parenting situations.

1. Which parts of you come up in different parenting situations, and what are their roles?
    - Example: "My organizer part takes over when it's time to get the kids ready for school, and my nurturing part comes out during bedtime."
    - Reflection: _____

Step 2: Understanding How These Parts Affect Your Parenting

- **Instructions**: Write down how these parts affect your relationship with your child. Do they help or hinder your ability to connect and lead from the Self?

1. How do your parenting parts impact your relationship with your child?
    - Reflection: _____

Step 3: Offering Compassion to Your Parenting Parts

- **Instructions**: Approach your parenting parts with compassion, acknowledging that they are trying to help you. Reflect on how you can balance their influence with Self-leadership.

1. How can you offer compassion to your parenting parts and bring more Self-leadership into your parenting?
    - Reflection: _____

Tips:

- Parenting involves many parts that play different roles. Recognizing these parts helps you understand how they affect your relationship with your child.
- Lead from your Self as much as possible, balancing your parenting parts with calm, compassionate leadership.

Therapist Comments/Feedback:

- "You're doing great work identifying your parenting parts. Keep balancing their roles with Self-leadership to strengthen your connection with your child."

Worksheet 136: Recognizing Your Child's Parts

Goal: To help parents recognize and understand the parts that show up in their children, fostering empathy and emotional support.

Step 1: Identifying Your Child's Parts

- **Instructions**: Think about a recent interaction with your child where they expressed strong emotions or behaviors. Write down which parts of your child might have been active and why.

1. What interaction did you have with your child, and which parts of them do you think were active?
    - Example: "My child's anxious part came up when we were about to leave for a new school."
    - Reflection: _____

Step 2: Understanding the Role of These Parts

- **Instructions**: Reflect on what these parts of your child were trying to accomplish or protect. Write down how you can approach these parts

1. What do you think your child's parts were trying to accomplish or protect during this interaction?
    - Example: "I think their anxious part was trying to protect them from feeling scared about the new school."
    - Reflection: _____

Step 3: Offering Compassion to Your Child's Parts

- **Instructions**: Approach your child's parts with compassion, recognizing that their behaviors and emotions are driven by internal needs. Write down how you can offer support and help soothe these parts.

1. How can you offer compassion and support to your child's parts, helping them feel safe and understood?
    - Reflection: _____

Tips:

- Recognizing your child's parts helps you understand their emotions and behaviors from a place of empathy. Approach them with curiosity, asking what their parts need.
- Encourage open communication with your child, allowing them to express their feelings in a safe environment.

Therapist Comments/Feedback:

- "Your awareness of your child's parts is a great step toward fostering a deeper emotional connection. Keep offering compassion and support, and you'll help them feel more secure."

Worksheet 137: Using Co-Regulation to Support Children

Goal: To help parents practice co-regulation with their children, teaching them how to support their emotional regulation by modeling calm and compassionate behavior.

Step 1: Recognizing When Co-Regulation Is Needed

- **Instructions**: Reflect on moments when your child's emotions seem overwhelming or out of control. Write down an example where co-regulation could help soothe their emotional state.

1. When did your child's emotions become overwhelming, and how could co-regulation help in this situation?
    - Example: "My child became upset when they couldn't finish a puzzle, and I could have helped them regulate by staying calm and guiding them through it."
    - Reflection: _____

Step 2: Practicing Co-Regulation

- **Instructions**: During the next emotional situation with your child, practice co-regulation by staying calm, breathing deeply, and modeling emotional regulation. Reflect on how your calm energy helped soothe your child.

1. How did practicing co-regulation with your child affect their emotional state?
    - Reflection: _____

Step 3: Reflecting on the Benefits of Co-Regulation

- **Instructions**: Write down how co-regulation improved the emotional atmosphere and how you plan to continue using it in future situations.

1. How has co-regulation improved your relationship with your child, and how will you incorporate it more regularly?
    - Reflection: _____

Tips:

- Co-regulation helps children learn how to regulate their emotions by mirroring your calm energy. Practice staying grounded and composed during your child's emotional moments.
- Use deep breathing and soothing tones to show your child how to stay calm in the face of frustration or stress.

Therapist Comments/Feedback:

- "Your use of co-regulation is a powerful tool for supporting your child's emotional development. Keep practicing this, and you'll see positive changes in how they manage their emotions."

Worksheet 138: Parenting with Compassion and Self-Leadership

Goal: To help parents lead from the Self in their parenting, promoting compassion, patience, and emotional connection with their children.

Step 1: Recognizing When to Lead from the Self

- **Instructions**: Reflect on a recent parenting moment where your parts took over instead of your Self. Write down what happened and which parts were active.

1. What parenting situation occurred, and which parts took over instead of your Self?
    - Example: "I felt frustrated when my child wasn't listening, and my impatient part took over."
    - Reflection: _____

Step 2: Leading from the Self in Future Situations

- **Instructions**: The next time you feel a parenting challenge arise, pause and connect with your Self before responding. Focus on leading with calm, compassion, and curiosity.

1. How did leading from your Self change the way you handled the parenting situation?
    - Reflection: _____

Step 3: Reflecting on the Impact of Self-Led Parenting

- **Instructions**: Write down how leading from your Self affected your relationship with your child and how you plan to continue practicing Self-leadership in your parenting.

1. How has Self-leadership improved your relationship with your child, and how will you continue practicing it?

- Reflection: _____

Tips:

- Parenting with Self-leadership requires mindfulness and patience. Pause before reacting and check in with your Self to ensure you're leading with compassion and understanding.
- Model emotional regulation and empathy for your children—they will learn from your example.

Therapist Comments/Feedback:

- "Leading from your Self in parenting is transformative. Keep practicing this approach, and it will strengthen your relationship with your child while fostering emotional safety and trust."

Part 18: Long-Term Healing and Growth

These worksheets in **Part 18: Long-Term Healing and Growth** are designed to guide users through a lifelong process of healing and self-leadership. By tracking progress, preventing burnout, and setting new goals for growth, these exercises help ensure that the healing journey is sustained and that emotional resilience and Self-leadership continue to deepen over time.

Tracking Your Healing Journey

Worksheet 139: Daily Check-In with Parts and Emotions

Goal: To help you regularly check in with your parts and emotions, promoting ongoing self-awareness and emotional balance.

Step 1: Identifying Active Parts

- **Instructions**: At the end of each day, take a few moments to reflect on which parts of you were most active. Write down which parts showed up and what emotions they carried.

1. Which parts were most active today, and what emotions did they carry?
    - Example: "My anxious part was active during the meeting, and it carried fear of failure."
    - Reflection: _____

Step 2: Reflecting on Your Emotional State

- **Instructions**: Reflect on how the emotions from your parts influenced your overall mood or behaviors throughout the day.

1. How did these emotions impact your mood and actions today?
    - Reflection: _____

Step 3: Offering Compassion to Parts

- **Instructions**: Approach your parts with compassion, recognizing their efforts to help you. Write down how you can offer understanding and support to these parts.

1. How can you offer compassion and support to your parts based on today's experiences?

- Reflection: _____

Tips:

- Daily check-ins help you stay connected to your parts and emotions, allowing for regular self-awareness and healing.
- Be consistent with this practice, even on days when emotions feel subtle or calm.

Therapist Comments/Feedback:

- "Your daily check-ins are a powerful way to stay in tune with your internal system. Keep offering compassion to your parts, and you'll notice a greater sense of emotional balance over time."

Worksheet 140: Monthly Reflection on Unburdening Progress

Goal: To help you reflect on your monthly progress with unburdening parts and healing emotional wounds.

Step 1: Reviewing Unburdening Work

- **Instructions**: Reflect on the past month and write down which parts went through the unburdening process. Note what emotional burdens were released.

1. Which parts went through unburdening this month, and what burdens were released?

    - Example: "My exile released the burden of shame from past experiences of rejection."
    - Reflection: _____

Step 2: Reflecting on Emotional Shifts

- **Instructions**: Write down how unburdening affected your emotional state and relationships over the past month. What shifts did you notice in your parts or overall well-being?

1. What emotional shifts have you noticed since unburdening these parts?
    - Reflection: _____

Step 3: Planning for Continued Healing

- **Instructions**: Based on your progress this month, write down your goals for the next phase of healing. What parts need continued attention, and how will you support them?

1. What are your healing goals for the upcoming month?
    - Reflection: _____

Tips:

- Monthly reflections give you the space to recognize your healing progress and plan for continued work with your parts.
- Acknowledge the emotional shifts you've experienced, even if they feel small—each step is progress.

Therapist Comments/Feedback:

- "You're making great strides with unburdening. Keep reflecting on your progress each month to stay connected to your healing journey."

Worksheet 141: Yearly Review of Growth in Self-Leadership

Goal: To help you reflect on your yearly growth in Self-leadership, recognizing how your ability to lead your parts has evolved.

Step 1: Reflecting on Self-Led Moments

- **Instructions**: Think about key moments from the past year where you led your parts from the Self. Write down examples where you handled challenges with calm, curiosity, and compassion.

1. What were some of the key moments where you led from the Self this year?
    - Example: "I stayed calm during a family argument and listened to my parts without letting them take over."
    - Reflection: _____

Step 2: Recognizing Growth in Self-Leadership

- **Instructions**: Write down how your ability to lead from the Self has grown over the past year. What changes have you noticed in how you respond to your parts and external challenges?

1. How has your Self-leadership grown over the past year, and what changes have you noticed?
    - Reflection: _____

Step 3: Setting Intentions for Future Growth

- **Instructions**: Based on your progress, write down your intentions for continuing to strengthen your Self-leadership in the coming year.

1. What are your intentions for further developing Self-leadership over the next year?
    - Reflection: _____

Tips:

- Self-leadership is a journey that evolves over time. Reflecting on yearly growth helps you see how far you've come and where you want to go.
- Celebrate the moments where you led from the Self, even if they seemed small—they are evidence of your progress.

Therapist Comments/Feedback:
- "Your reflection on Self-leadership shows incredible growth. Keep setting goals for future development, and you'll continue to strengthen your ability to lead with compassion and calm."

Worksheet 142: Goals for Continued Healing

Goal: To help you set clear goals for ongoing healing, ensuring that you continue to support your parts and deepen your self-awareness.

Step 1: Reflecting on Current Healing Needs

- **Instructions**: Reflect on where you are in your healing journey and write down which parts still need attention or support.

1. Which parts of your system need further healing or support?
   - Example: "My perfectionist part still feels anxious about failure and needs more compassion."
   - Reflection: _____

Step 2: Setting Clear Healing Goals

- **Instructions**: Write down specific goals for how you will continue to support these parts and deepen your healing over the next few months.

1. What are your goals for continuing your healing journey, and how will you support your parts?

- o   Reflection: _____

Step 3: Creating a Plan for Healing

- **Instructions**: Create a plan for achieving these goals, outlining what steps you will take, such as continuing unburdening work, practicing mindfulness, or seeking additional support.

1. What steps will you take to achieve your healing goals?
    - o   Reflection: _____

Tips:

- Setting clear healing goals helps you stay focused and committed to your ongoing growth. Be specific about what steps you'll take to support your parts.
- Revisit these goals regularly to assess your progress and make adjustments as needed.

Therapist Comments/Feedback:

- "Your healing goals show a strong commitment to ongoing growth. Keep revisiting these goals to stay connected to your parts and ensure continued progress."

Sustaining Self-Leadership

Worksheet 143: Weekly Practices to Stay Connected to the Self
Goal: To help you develop weekly practices that keep you connected to your Self, ensuring that you lead your internal system with calm and compassion.

Step 1: Identifying Practices That Support Self-Connection

- **Instructions**: Write down weekly practices that help you stay connected to your Self. These could include mindfulness, journaling, or regular check-ins with your parts.

1. What weekly practices will help you stay connected to your Self?
    - Example: "I will practice 10 minutes of mindfulness each morning and journal about my parts on Sunday evenings."
    - Reflection: _____

Step 2: Creating a Weekly Routine

- **Instructions**: Write down how you will incorporate these practices into your weekly routine. Be specific about when and how you will engage with them.

1. How will you incorporate these practices into your weekly routine?
    - Reflection: _____

Step 3: Reflecting on the Benefits of Self-Connection

- **Instructions**: Reflect on how these weekly practices help you stay grounded and connected to your Self, ensuring that you lead from a place of calm and compassion.

1. How have these weekly practices helped you stay connected to your Self?
    - Reflection: _____

Tips:

- Weekly practices are essential for maintaining a connection to your Self. Choose practices that resonate with you and fit into your routine.

- Consistency is key—commit to these practices even when life gets busy or stressful.

Therapist Comments/Feedback:

- "Your commitment to weekly practices shows a deep dedication to staying connected to your Self. Keep up these routines, and they will support your long-term healing and growth."

Worksheet 144: How to Reconnect with Parts After a Relapse

Goal: To guide you through reconnecting with your parts after a relapse or setback, helping you restore balance and self-compassion.

Step 1: Reflecting on the Relapse

- **Instructions**: Think about a recent relapse where parts took over and led to behaviors or emotions that felt overwhelming. Write down which parts were involved and what triggered the relapse.

1. What relapse occurred, and which parts were involved?
    - Example: "My firefighter part took over, and I coped by avoiding responsibilities for a few days."
    - Reflection: _____

Step 2: Reconnecting with Parts After the Relapse

- **Instructions**: Approach your parts with compassion and curiosity. Write down how you can reconnect with the parts that were active during the relapse. What do they need from you to feel supported and understood?

1. How can you reconnect with these parts, and what do they need to feel supported?

- Example: "I can reconnect with my firefighter part by listening to its fears and offering it compassion instead of judgment."
- Reflection: _____

Step 3: Restoring Balance in the System

- **Instructions**: Reflect on how you can bring your system back into balance after the relapse. Write down how you can offer compassion to all your parts and return to Self-leadership.

1. How can you restore balance in your system and lead from the Self after the relapse?
   - Reflection: _____

Tips:

- Relapses are a normal part of the healing journey. Approach them with curiosity and compassion rather than self-criticism.
- Use relapses as an opportunity to learn more about your parts and what they need for continued healing.

Therapist Comments/Feedback:

- "It's important to approach relapses with self-compassion. By reconnecting with your parts and restoring balance, you can continue your healing without feeling discouraged."

Worksheet 145: Preventing Burnout When Leading from the Self

Goal: To help you prevent burnout while leading from the Self, ensuring that you maintain emotional resilience and balance.

Step 1: Identifying Signs of Burnout

- **Instructions**: Reflect on times when you felt emotionally exhausted or disconnected from your Self. Write down the signs of burnout you noticed and how it affected your internal system.

1. What signs of burnout have you experienced, and how did they affect your ability to lead from the Self?
    - Example: "I felt overwhelmed and disconnected from my parts, which led to frustration and withdrawal."
    - Reflection: _____

Step 2: Creating a Burnout Prevention Plan

- **Instructions**: Write down strategies you can use to prevent burnout. These might include setting boundaries, practicing self-care, or delegating tasks to your parts to ensure balance.

1. What strategies will you use to prevent burnout and maintain emotional resilience?
    - Reflection: _____

Step 3: Reflecting on Balance in Self-Leadership

- **Instructions**: Reflect on how maintaining a balance between Self-leadership and rest will help you sustain your emotional well-being. Write down your plan for ensuring this balance.

1. How will you balance leading from the Self with rest and self-care to prevent burnout?
    - Reflection: _____

Tips:

- Burnout can happen when you take on too much responsibility without rest. Make sure to delegate tasks to your parts and practice self-care.
- Regularly check in with your parts and ensure that you're not overextending yourself emotionally.

Therapist Comments/Feedback:

- "Preventing burnout is crucial to sustaining Self-leadership. Keep balancing your responsibilities with self-care to maintain emotional resilience and avoid exhaustion."

Worksheet 146: Creating a Plan for Continued Self-Growth

Goal: To help you create a personalized plan for ongoing self-growth, ensuring that you continue to evolve in your healing journey.

Step 1: Reflecting on Current Areas of Growth

- **Instructions**: Reflect on your current healing journey and write down the areas where you've grown the most. Identify the parts of your internal system that have healed or strengthened.

1. What areas of your healing journey have shown the most growth, and how have you evolved?
    - Example: "I've become more compassionate toward my perfectionist part, and I've learned to soothe it without letting it take over."
    - Reflection: _____

Step 2: Setting Goals for Future Growth

- **Instructions**: Write down specific goals for continued self-growth. These could include deepening your Self-leadership, healing more parts, or enhancing your mindfulness practice.

1. What are your goals for continued self-growth, and how will you achieve them?
    - Reflection: _____

Step 3: Creating a Growth Plan

- **Instructions**: Create a plan for how you will achieve your goals. Outline the steps you'll take, such as working with specific parts, practicing mindfulness, or seeking additional support.

1. What steps will you take to ensure your continued growth in healing and Self-leadership?
    - Reflection: _____

Tips:

- Continued growth requires ongoing self-reflection and a willingness to set new goals. Be clear about the areas you want to work on and the steps you'll take to get there.
- Celebrate your progress along the way, and recognize that growth is a lifelong journey.

Therapist Comments/Feedback:

- "Your commitment to ongoing growth is inspiring. Keep setting goals for self-improvement and following through with your plan to continue evolving in your healing journey."

Worksheet 147: Recognizing Patterns in Your Healing Journey

Goal: To help you identify recurring patterns in your healing journey, allowing you to gain deeper insights into your growth and challenges.

Step 1: Identifying Patterns

- **Instructions**: Reflect on your healing journey and write down any patterns you've noticed in how your parts react to certain situations. These could be emotional triggers, behaviors, or protective responses that recur over time.

1. What patterns have you noticed in your healing journey, and how do they affect your internal system?
    - Example: "My perfectionist part gets activated whenever I take on a new project, and it leads to anxiety."
    - Reflection: _____

Step 2: Understanding the Impact of These Patterns

- **Instructions**: Write down how these patterns have impacted your healing progress. Have they slowed down your growth, or have they brought awareness to areas that need more attention?

1. How have these patterns affected your healing progress, and what have you learned from them?
    - Reflection: _____

Step 3: Creating a Plan to Address Patterns

- **Instructions**: Based on the patterns you've identified, write down a plan for addressing them in the future. What strategies will you use to interrupt these patterns and bring more Self-leadership to these situations?

1. What steps will you take to address recurring patterns and lead from your Self in these situations?
    - Reflection: _____

Tips:

- Recognizing patterns in your healing journey allows you to break cycles and make conscious choices about how you respond to triggers.
- Use these insights to develop new strategies that bring more awareness and balance to your internal system.

Therapist Comments/Feedback:

- "Identifying patterns is an important part of self-awareness. By recognizing and addressing these patterns, you'll be able to make more conscious choices about how you lead your parts."

Worksheet 148: Building Emotional Resilience for Future Challenges

Goal: To help you strengthen emotional resilience, preparing you to navigate future challenges with more confidence and balance.

Step 1: Reflecting on Past Challenges

- **Instructions**: Think about a recent challenge or emotionally difficult situation. Write down which parts of you were activated and how you responded to the challenge.

1. What recent challenge did you face, and which parts were activated during that time?

- Example: "I faced a major deadline at work, and my anxious part took over, leading to stress and frustration."
- Reflection: _____

Step 2: Learning from the Challenge

- **Instructions**: Reflect on how you handled the challenge. What did you learn about your parts, and how could you have responded differently from the Self?

1. What did you learn about your parts from this challenge, and how could you have responded with more Self-leadership?
    - Reflection: _____

Step 3: Strengthening Resilience for Future Challenges

- **Instructions**: Write down steps you will take to build emotional resilience for future challenges. This could include practicing mindfulness, strengthening Self-leadership, or developing new coping strategies.

1. What steps will you take to strengthen your emotional resilience for future challenges?
    - Reflection: _____

Tips:

- Emotional resilience is built through reflection and practice. Use each challenge as an opportunity to learn more about your parts and how to respond with greater balance.
- Strengthening Self-leadership in challenging times helps create more emotional stability in your internal system.

Therapist Comments/Feedback:

- "Building resilience is key to navigating life's challenges. By reflecting on past difficulties and developing new strategies, you're preparing yourself to handle future challenges with more ease."

Worksheet 149: Evaluating Your Relationship with Self-Compassion

Goal: To help you evaluate your relationship with self-compassion, ensuring that you are offering yourself kindness and understanding throughout your healing journey.

Step 1: Reflecting on Your Self-Compassion Practices

- **Instructions**: Think about how often you practice self-compassion. Write down examples of times when you've been kind to yourself and moments when you've been critical.

1. How often do you practice self-compassion, and what are some examples of kindness or criticism toward yourself?
    - Example: "I'm kind to myself when I make small mistakes, but I tend to be critical when I feel like I've let others down."
    - Reflection: _____

Step 2: Understanding the Impact of Self-Compassion

- **Instructions**: Write down how practicing self-compassion affects your emotional well-being and healing progress. How does being critical or kind to yourself influence your parts and overall system?

1. How does self-compassion (or a lack of it) impact your emotional well-being and healing progress?
    - Reflection: _____

Step 3: Creating a Plan to Strengthen Self-Compassion

- **Instructions**: Write down steps you will take to strengthen your self-compassion practice. What daily or weekly actions can you implement to ensure you are offering yourself more kindness?

1. What steps will you take to strengthen your self-compassion practice?
    - Reflection: _____

Tips:

- Self-compassion is essential for healing. Regularly check in with how kind or critical you are toward yourself, and make conscious efforts to offer yourself more understanding.
- Practice self-compassion daily, especially during moments of difficulty or when you feel disappointed in yourself.

Therapist Comments/Feedback:

- "Your relationship with self-compassion is crucial to your overall healing. By strengthening this practice, you'll create more space for emotional growth and resilience."

Worksheet 150: Cultivating Gratitude in Your Healing Journey

Goal: To help you cultivate gratitude for your healing journey and the progress you've made, fostering a positive outlook on your growth.

Step 1: Reflecting on Your Healing Journey

- **Instructions**: Take time to reflect on how far you've come in your healing journey. Write down specific moments or milestones where you've made progress, no matter how small.

1. What milestones or moments of progress have you experienced in your healing journey?
    - Example: "I've learned to manage my anxious part with more compassion, and I've become more patient with myself."
    - Reflection: _____

Step 2: Practicing Gratitude for Your Parts

- **Instructions**: Write down how you can express gratitude toward your parts for their roles in your healing. Even protective parts that may seem challenging have been working to support you.

1. How can you express gratitude to your parts for their roles in your healing journey?
    - Reflection: _____

Step 3: Reflecting on Gratitude's Impact on Healing

- **Instructions**: Reflect on how practicing gratitude toward yourself and your parts can enhance your healing journey. Write down how gratitude has affected your emotional state and outlook on healing.

1. How has practicing gratitude toward your parts and healing journey impacted your emotions and mindset?
    - Reflection: _____

Tips:

- Gratitude is a powerful tool for shifting your mindset and fostering positivity. Take time each day or week to reflect on the progress you've made and express gratitude for your parts.
- Even small milestones are worth celebrating, as they show that you are moving forward in your healing journey.

Therapist Comments/Feedback:

- "Cultivating gratitude for your healing journey helps shift your focus to the positive progress you've made. Keep practicing gratitude regularly to enhance your emotional well-being."

Conclusion

As you reach the conclusion of **"The Internal Family Systems Therapy Worksheets: 150 Guided Essential Tools for Emotional Healing, Self-Leadership, and Personal Growth,"** it's essential to acknowledge the profound journey you've undertaken. Internal Family Systems (IFS) therapy offers not only a path to understanding your inner world but also a transformative approach to healing and integrating the various parts that make up your internal system. Each part—whether a protector, manager, firefighter, or exile—holds its own unique story, emotions, and needs, and your ability to engage with them through the exercises in this workbook marks a significant step toward wholeness.

Throughout this workbook, you have explored many critical aspects of IFS, from identifying the protector parts that manage your day-to-day experiences to delving into the deep wounds carried by your exiled parts. You've unburdened old emotions, soothed anxious and overwhelmed parts, and, perhaps most importantly, strengthened your relationship with your Self—the calm, compassionate, and wise leader within you. Each worksheet has been designed to guide you in building self-awareness, emotional resilience, and Self-leadership, equipping you with the tools to navigate life's complexities with greater clarity and balance.

Reflecting on Your Healing Journey

Healing through IFS is not a linear process, nor is it one that can be rushed. Every step you've taken has helped you peel back layers of emotional defenses and address the underlying wounds that your parts have carried for years, or even decades. Some of the worksheets may have guided you through particularly difficult terrain—exploring deeply entrenched fears, past traumas, or relationship conflicts. But through these challenges, you've also had the opportunity to meet your parts with compassion, to listen to their concerns, and to understand their roles within your system.

At the heart of IFS is the concept of the Self—a powerful, compassionate presence that can lead your internal system toward healing and balance. This workbook has been your guide in not only understanding your parts but also in learning how to access and embody your Self. With Self-leadership, you have begun to foster a sense of peace, harmony, and internal cooperation, allowing each of your parts to feel seen, heard, and understood.

As you reflect on your progress, take pride in the courage it took to engage with these parts, some of which may have been exiled or burdened for a long time. The act of showing up for your parts, of listening to their needs, and of unburdening them from the weight of past pain, is a profound act of healing. Through this work, you have not only gained insight into your internal system but also made space for growth, transformation, and personal empowerment.

The Long-Term Value of Self-Leadership

One of the core goals of this workbook is to help you cultivate Self-leadership, a vital component in long-term emotional well-being. Self-leadership means learning how to respond to life's challenges from a place of calm, clarity, and compassion, rather than from the reactive place of wounded or protective parts. It's about stepping into your life with a deep sense of inner authority, knowing that you are capable of leading your parts through any conflict, emotional trigger, or difficult decision.

Self-leadership is an ongoing practice, one that requires regular attention and care. The worksheets in this book have given you structured opportunities to practice Self-leadership in different contexts—whether dealing with anxiety, managing relationship conflicts, healing trauma, or simply checking in with your parts on a daily basis. As you continue on this journey, remember that Self-leadership is not about perfection, but about presence. It's about being there for your parts, especially when things feel difficult or overwhelming, and guiding them with the compassion and wisdom of your Self.

Sustaining Healing and Growth

Healing through IFS is not a destination but a lifelong process. The work you've done with this workbook has laid a strong foundation for continued personal growth and healing, but it's essential to remember that the process of self-discovery and emotional healing evolves over time. New challenges may arise, new parts may surface, or old burdens may reappear—but with the skills and tools you've developed through this workbook, you are better equipped to handle these challenges.

The worksheets dedicated to long-term growth and emotional resilience are there to support you in this ongoing process. Tools like the **Daily Check-In with Parts and Emotions** worksheet, **Monthly Reflection on Unburdening Progress**, and **Yearly Review of Growth in Self-Leadership** are designed to help you stay engaged with your internal system, track your progress, and set new goals for continued healing.

These worksheets offer you the structure to reflect on your journey, set intentions for future growth, and remain connected to your parts in a healthy and balanced way. Use them as a regular practice to prevent emotional stagnation, burnout, or regression. By maintaining an active relationship with your parts and practicing Self-leadership daily, you will continue to grow emotionally, expand your self-awareness, and sustain the healing you've worked so hard to achieve.

Applying IFS in Your Life

The exercises in this book have guided you through a variety of emotional challenges, from dealing with anxiety and trauma to improving relationships and parenting with compassion. Now, the challenge is to apply the lessons and insights gained from these worksheets in your daily life.

In your relationships, for example, practicing the tools from the **IFS for Couples** and **IFS for Parenting** sections can help you navigate conflict with greater understanding and compassion. When triggered by a loved one's behavior, remember to check in with your parts before reacting, and to lead the conversation from your Self. In moments of stress or overwhelm, revisit the exercises on soothing anxious parts and bringing calm to your internal system. These skills are not just for your personal healing—they are essential tools for improving your relationships with others and fostering emotional safety in your interactions.

Moreover, as life presents new challenges—whether in your personal relationships, professional life, or emotional health—you now have the resources to lead yourself through these difficulties with clarity, confidence, and compassion. The Self-led practices, unburdening techniques, and mindfulness exercises you've learned here are powerful tools for managing stress, resolving conflict, and preventing emotional overwhelm.

Looking Forward

As you move forward, take with you the knowledge that healing is not a one-time event but an ongoing journey. Each part of you—whether a protector, an exile, or a manager—deserves your attention and care, and you now have the tools to offer them the compassion and understanding they need. Keep checking in with your internal system regularly, continue building relationships with your parts, and, most importantly, trust in your Self to guide you through whatever life may bring.

This workbook is here as a resource whenever you need it. Revisit the worksheets, practice the exercises, and remember that the work of emotional healing and personal growth is a lifelong commitment. The transformation you've already experienced is a testament to the power of IFS and your willingness to engage in this deep work.

Thank you for embarking on this journey and trusting in the process of Internal Family Systems therapy. May you continue to grow in Self-leadership, healing, and personal transformation, and may you always find peace, clarity, and compassion in the presence of your Self.

Reference

1. Haddock, S.A., Weiler, L.M., Trump, L.J., & Henry, K.L., 2016. The efficacy of Internal Family Systems therapy in the treatment of depression among female college students: A pilot study. *Journal of Marital and Family Therapy*, 42(1), pp.175–189.

2. Hodgdon, H., 2021. Internal Family Systems (IFS) therapy for post-traumatic stress disorder (PTSD) among survivors of multiple childhood trauma: A pilot effectiveness study. *Journal of Aggression, Maltreatment & Trauma*, 30(6), pp.723–739.

3. Shadick, N.A., et al., 2013. A randomized controlled trial of an Internal Family Systems-based psychotherapeutic intervention on outcomes in rheumatoid arthritis: A proof-of-concept study. *The Journal of Rheumatology*, 40(7), pp.1025-1032.

4. Schwartz, R.C., 2020. Internal Family Systems (IFS) therapy for post-traumatic stress disorder: A new approach. *Journal of Trauma & Dissociation*, 21(3), pp.251-268.

5. Anderson, F.G., Sweezy, M., & Schwartz, R.C., 2017. Internal Family Systems skills training manual: Trauma-informed treatment. PESI Publishing.

6. Lucero, R., Jones, A.C., & Hunsaker, J.C., 2018. Using Internal Family Systems theory in the treatment of combat veterans with post-traumatic stress disorder and their families. *Contemporary Family Therapy*, 40(3), pp.266–275.

7. Huh, H.J., Kim, S.Y., Yu, J.J., & Chae, J.H., 2014. Childhood trauma and adult interpersonal relationship problems in patients with depression and anxiety disorders. *Annals of General Psychiatry*, 13(1), pp.26-33.

8. Mithoefer, M.C., et al., 2019. MDMA-assisted psychotherapy for PTSD: A randomized, double-blind, placebo-controlled phase 3 study. *Lancet Psychiatry*, 6(8), pp.735-746.

9. MacIntosh, H., Fletcher, K., & Collin-Vézina, D., 2016. "I was like damaged, used goods": Thematic analysis of disclosures of childhood sexual abuse to romantic partners. *Marriage and Family Review*, 52(6), pp.598-611.

10. Kim, J.S., 2008. Examining the effectiveness of solution-focused brief therapy: A meta-analysis. *Research on Social Work Practice*, 18(2), pp.107–116.

11. Schwartz, R.C., & Sweezy, M., 2019. The evolution of Internal Family Systems therapy. *Journal of Marital and Family Therapy*, 45(1), pp.22-35.

12. Patel, M., Skelton, K., & Kelly, U., 2011. Interpersonal violence, PTSD, and mental health in women veterans. *Research in Nursing & Health*, 34(6), pp.457–467.

13. McLean, I.A., 2013. The male victim of sexual assault. *Best Practice & Research Clinical Obstetrics & Gynaecology*, 27(1), pp.39–46.

14. Kessler, R.C., et al., 2017. Trauma and PTSD in the WHO world mental health surveys. *European Journal of Psychotraumatology*, 8(5), p.1353383.

15. Koss, M.P., et al., 2007. Revising the SES: A collaborative process to improve assessment of sexual aggression and victimization. *Psychology of Women Quarterly*, 31(4), pp.357–370.

16. Kilpatrick, D.G., et al., 2013. National estimates of exposure to traumatic events and PTSD prevalence using DSM-IV and DSM-5 criteria. *Journal of Traumatic Stress*, 26(5), pp.537–547.

17. Kia-Keating, M., Sorsoli, L., & Grossman, F.K., 2010. Relational challenges and recovery processes in male survivors of childhood sexual abuse. *Journal of Interpersonal Violence*, 25(4), pp.666–683.

18. Mithoefer, M.C., et al., 2016. MDMA-assisted psychotherapy for PTSD: Long-term follow-up results from phase 2 trials. *Journal of Psychopharmacology*, 30(12), pp.1228–1238.

19. Schwartz, R.C., 2013. The legacy of family therapy and the future of Internal Family Systems. *Journal of Family Therapy*, 35(3), pp.229-244.

20. Schwartz, R.C., 2001. The Internal Family Systems model. *Psychotherapy Networker*, 25(3), pp.36-41.

21. Schwartz, R.C., & Goulding, R., 2017. Family systems theory and its relationship to IFS. *Journal of Family Process*, 56(2), pp.212-228.

22. Haddock, S.A., 2018. Efficacy of IFS therapy in college students. *Journal of Marital and Family Therapy*, 44(3), pp.234–247.

23. Meston, C.M., Rellini, A.H., & Heiman, J.R., 2006. Women's history of sexual abuse, their sexuality, and sexual self-schemas. *Journal of Consulting and Clinical Psychology*, 74(2), pp.229-236.

24. Maltz, W., 2012. The sexual healing journey: A guide for survivors of sexual abuse. William Morrow.

25. Lucero, R., Jones, A.C., & Hunsaker, J.C., 2019. Veterans with PTSD and Internal Family Systems. *Journal of Family Therapy*, 41(2), pp.134-147.

26. Anderson, F.G., 2021. Transcending trauma: Healing complex PTSD with Internal Family Systems. PESI Publishing.

27. Ford, J.D., Courtois, C.A., Steele, K., & Van der Kolk, B.A., 2016. Treating complex trauma: A sequenced, relationship-based approach. *Journal of Traumatic Stress*, 29(1), pp.20–28.

28. Shadick, N.A., et al., 2017. Internal Family Systems therapy reduces pain in rheumatoid arthritis: A pilot study. *Rheumatology*, 56(5), pp.1234-1241.

v.ingramcontent.com/pod-product-compliance
ning Source LLC
ersburg PA
80552090426
B00016B/3210